Oklahoma Notes

Embryology

Second Edition

Robert E. Coalson
James J. Tomasek

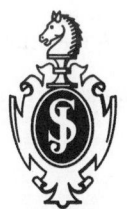

Springer-Verlag
New York Berlin Heidelberg London Paris
Tokyo Hong Kong Barcelona Budapest

Robert E. Coalson, Ph.D.
James J. Tomasek, Ph.D.
Department of Anatomical Sciences
College of Medicine
Health Sciences Center
The University of Oklahoma
Oklahoma City, OK 73190
USA

Library of Congress Cataloging-in-Publication Data
Coalson, Robert E.
    Embryology / Robert E. Coalson, James J. Tomasek—2nd ed.
      p.   cm.—(Oklahoma notes)

    1. Embryology, Human—Outlines, syllabi, etc.
    2. Embryology, Human—Examinations, questions, etc.
    I. Tomasek, James J.   II. Title.   III. Series.
      [DNLM: 1. Embryology—examination questions.
    2. Embryology—outlines.   QS 18 C652eb]
    QM601L64   1992
    612.6′4′ 0076—dc20
    DNLM/DLC
    for Library of Congress   92-2136

Printed on acid-free paper.

Production managed by Henry Krell; manufacturing supervised by Jacqui Ashri.
Camera-ready copy prepared by the authors.

9 8 7 6 5 4 3 2 1

ISBN-13: 978-0-387-97776-8   e-ISBN-13: 978-1-4612-2900-1
DOI: 10.1007/ 978-1-4612-2900-1

Preface to the
Oklahoma Notes

In 1973, the University of Oklahoma College of Medicine instituted a requirement for passage of the Part 1 National Boards for promotion to the third year. To assist students in preparation for this examination, a two-week review of the basic sciences was added to the curriculum in 1975. Ten review texts were written by the faculty: four in anatomical sciences and one each in the other six basic sciences. Self-instructional quizzes were also developed by each discipline and administered during the review period.

The first year the course was instituted the Total Score performance on National Boards Part I increased 60 points, with the relative standing of the school changing from 56th to 9th in the nation. The performance of the class since then has remained near the national candidate mean (500) with a range of 467 to 537. This improvement in our own students' performance has been documented (Hyde et al: Performance on NBME Part I examination in relation to policies regarding use of test. J. Med. Educ. 60:439–443, 1985).

A questionnaire was administered to one of the classes after they had completed the Boards; 82% rated the review books as the most beneficial part of the course. These texts were subsequently rewritten and made available for use by all students of medicine who were preparing for comprehensive examinations in the Basic Medical Sciences. Since their introduction in 1987, over a quarter of a million copies have been sold. Assuming that 60,000 students have been first-time takers in the intervening five years, this equates to an average of four books per examinee.

Obviously these texts have proven to be of value. The main reason is that they present a *concise overview* of each discipline, emphasizing the content and concepts most appropriate to the task at hand, i.e., passage of a comprehensive examination over the Basic Medical Sciences.

The recent changes in the licensure examination structure that have been made to create a Step 1/Step 2 process have necessitated a complete revision of the Oklahoma Notes. This task was begun in the summer of 1991; the book you are now holding is a product of that revision. Besides bringing each book up to date, the authors have made every effort to make the texts and review questions conform to the new format of the National Board of Medical Examiners tests.

I hope you will find these review books valuable in your preparation for the licensure exams. Good Luck!

Richard M. Hyde, Ph.D.
Executive Editor

Preface

This book was prepared to present an integrated review of selected topics in Human Embryology. It is designed specifically for students who completed standard courses in the various anatomical disciplines and who wish to review the developmental history of the major organ systems.

This book will provide medical students with a highly suitable review for Step 1 of the United States Medical Licensing Exam (USMLE, Step 1).

R. E. Coalson
J. J. Tomasek

Acknowledgments

We wish to acknowledge the invaluable assistance provided by our colleagues at the University of Oklahoma Health Sciences Center during preparation of this review. In particular, we would like to thank Ms. Nancy Halliday for proofreading, Mr. Shawn Schlinke for preparation of the illustrations, Mr. Melville Vaughan for assistance with mounting the illustrations, and Ms. Trenda Tanner for assistance with the typing.

Contents

CHAPTER 1: GAMETOGENESIS

CELLS AND CHROMOSOMES

DIPLOID CELLS

In humans, the cells comprising all renewing cell populations (including the precursors of germ cells) are **diploid** (2N) and possess a total of 46 chromosomes. When the chromosomes of dividing cells are **karyotyped**, it can be determined that, with one exception (in males), they occur in pairs which are morphologically identical, i.e., **homologous**. One member of each homologous pair is of maternal origin, the other, its homologue, is of paternal origin. The numbers one through 22 are used to designate the **autosomal** (non-sex) chromosome pairs; the 23rd pair is referred to simply as the **sex chromosomes**. In females (46,XX) the maternal and paternal sex chromosomes are morphologically identical and are homologous like the autosomal chromosome pairs. In males (46,XY), the maternal (X-chromosome) and paternal (Y-chromosome) sex chromosomes are not identical morphologically and are, therefore, **nonhomologous**. The nonhomologous condition of the sex chromosomes in males provides the only instance in which the parental origin of a particular chromosome can be determined readily; this distinction is possible because the Y-chromosome is always derived from the father and the X-chromosome is always derived from the mother.

$$
\begin{aligned}
\text{diploid (2N) chromosome number} &= 46 \\
\text{autosomal chromosomes} &= 44 \text{ (22 homologous pairs)} \\
\text{sex chromosomes} &= 2 \\
\text{females} &= \text{XX (homologous)} \\
\text{males} &= \text{XY (nonhomologous)}
\end{aligned}
$$

HAPLOID CELLS (GAMETES)

The gametes (sperm and ova) are highly specialized reproductive cells containing only one-half (N or 23) the number of chromosomes found in renewing cell populations. The reduction in chromosome number is accomplished by two specialized cell cycles which are referred to as **Meiosis I and Meiosis II.**

$$
\begin{aligned}
\text{haploid (N) chromosome number} &= 23 \\
\text{autosomal chromosomes} &= 22 \text{ (one member from each pair)} \\
\text{sex chromosomes} &= 1 \\
\text{females} &= \text{X (always)} \\
\text{males} &= \text{X or Y}
\end{aligned}
$$

When two haploid gametes fuse at the time of fertilization, the diploid number of chromosomes is restored in the **zygote**.

CHROMOSOME MORPHOLOGY

Structurally, the chromosomes exhibit two characteristic areas or regions which are referred to as the **centromere** and the **arms**. The position of the centromere, which determines the relative lengths of the arms, is remarkably constant for each chromosome and is one of the major characteristics used to group chromosomes during karyotyping. Other techniques employed by cytogenetics laboratories, e.g., banding pattern in the arms, allow precise identification of all chromosomes within each

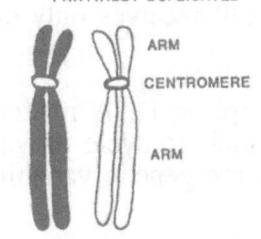

HOMOLOGOUS CHROMOSOMES
PARTIALLY DUPLICATED

ARM
CENTROMERE
ARM

EARLY METAPHASE
2 CHROMATIDS PER CHROMOSOME

karyotype group. Banding patterns are useful for detecting translocations, deletions and duplications affecting individual chromosomes.

CHROMOSOME DUPLICATION

It is important to remember that when the chromosomes are duplicated in preparation for cell division, that duplication of the arms and centromeres occurs during different periods (and phases) of the cell cycle.

Arm duplication (primarily DNA replication) always occurs during the S-phase of the intermitotic (interphase) period.

Centromeric duplication (division) always occurs during late metaphase of the mitotic period.

During prophase of the mitotic period, when chromosome condensation is well advanced, it can be determined easily that each chromosome consists of a single centromere uniting the duplicated arms. The two halves of each partially duplicated chromosome are called **chromatids**; chromatids become complete independent chromosomes only when each possesses its own centromere, i.e., during late metaphase.

FACTORS REGULATING DIPLOID AND HAPLOID (GAMETE) PRODUCTION

DIPLOID CELLS

The two most important events occurring during the regular mitotic cell cycles of diploid cells are DNA replication (interphase) and centromeric division (late metaphase). When both events (DNA replication and centromeric division) occur during the **same** cell cycle, the number of chromosomes in both daughter cells will remain constant (diploid) and the daughter cells will be identical genetically.

Coupling DNA replication and centromeric division within the same cell cycle provides the basic mechanism for maintaining the diploid chromosome number and genetic uniformity in the stem cells of all renewing cell populations including the precursors of germ cells.

HAPLOID CELLS (GAMETES)

During the two specialized cell cycles of gametogenesis (Meiosis I and Meiosis II), DNA replication and centromeric division occur in separate cell cycles. DNA replication occurs during meiosis I; centromeric division occurs during meiosis II. When cells divide without centromeric division, the number of chromosomes transmitted to daughter cells must be reduced by one-half. The resulting haploid daughter cells will **NOT** be genetically identical because each cell receives only one member (maternal or paternal) from each of the 23 chromosome pairs.

Uncoupling DNA replication and centromeric division so that only one event occurs during each meiotic cycle provides the basic mechanism for reducing chromosome number and for providing genetic variability among germs cells.

Meiosis I. Cells (future gametes) derived from the renewing population of gonial stem cells enter meiosis I as **diploid primary gametocytes** possessing 46 independent chromosomes. After cell division, the daughter cells leave meiosis I as **haploid secondary gametocytes** containing 23 partially duplicated chromosomes.

Interphase I. DNA replication by the entering primary gametocyte prepares it for the approaching cell division. After DNA replication the primary gametocyte is still diploid because its 46 chromosomes have only undergone arm duplication and have not duplicated their centromeres. **Note:** Shortly after DNA replication but before chromosome condensation is well advanced, the homologous chromosomes undergo **synapsis** and exchange genetic material **(crossing-over).** This unusual phenomenon occurs only during meiosis I and is one of the mechanisms provided to ensure genetic variability among gametes.

Metaphase I. Centromeric division does not occur and as a consequence, the daughter secondary gametocytes will receive only one-half (23) of the partially duplicated chromosomes. **Note:** Because the change from diploid to haploid chromosome number occurs at this time, the first meiotic division is called the **reduction division.**

The daughter, secondary gametocytes are **NOT** genetically identical because each cell receives only one member (maternal or paternal) from each chromosome pair and for each homologous pair, the chromosome distribution between daughter cells is random, i.e., **independent assortment of chromosomes.** The random assortment of chromosomes provides another mechanism for ensuring genetic variability among gametes.

Meiosis II. Cells enter meiosis II as haploid secondary gametocytes containing 23 partially duplicated chromosomes. After division, daughter cells leave as haploid 'tid cells' possessing 23 independent chromosomes.

Interphase II. DNA replication does **NOT** occur in secondary gametocytes because its 23 chromosomes are already partially duplicated.

Metaphase II. Centromeric division occurs during late metaphase and allows the 2 chromatids comprising each of the 23 partially duplicated chromosomes to separate as independent chromosomes for distribution to the daughter 'tid cells', i.e., 23 chromosomes per cell.

The daughter 'tid cells' are **NOT** genetically identical because of the crossing-over that occurred during interphase I.

Note: Unlike DNA replication, the biochemical events surrounding centromeric division are poorly understood. Centromeric division occurs very rapidly during late metaphase and appears to be effected simultaneously (or almost simultaneously) in all chromosomes during regular mitotic cycles and during meiosis II. Although the mechanism for synchronization is not known, the results of asynchronous division (nondisjunction and aneuploid) are well known and will be discussed later.

4

DURATION OF GAMETOGENESIS

In **males**, gametogenesis begins at puberty and continues into advanced age. Thymidine labeling indicates that the time required to produce mature sperm after the last replication of DNA by a primary spermatocyte during meiosis I is approximately 64 days.

In **females**, gametogenesis begins during late fetal life when all oogonia enter meiosis I and undergo their last replication of DNA. At birth the ovary contains only primary oocytes (with partially duplicated chromosomes) arrested in early

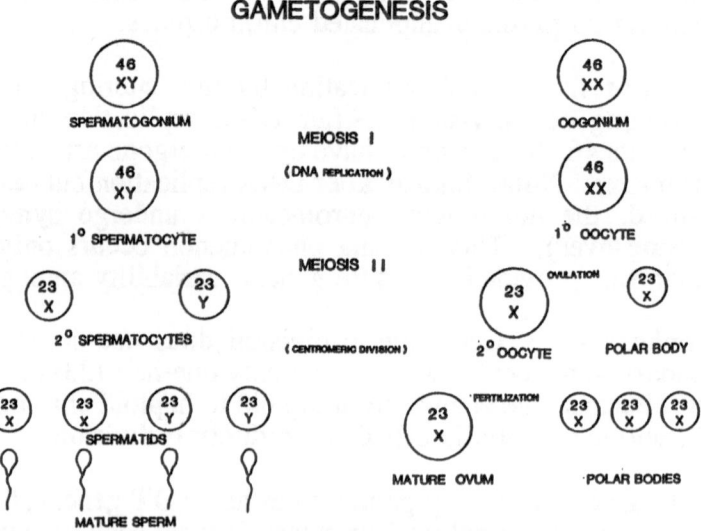

GAMETOGENESIS

prophase of meiosis I; meiosis I is completed many years later at the time of ovulation. The secondary oocyte completes meiosis II only at the time of fertilization. Consequently, the time required to produce a mature ovum from an oogonium may be as long as 40-45 years; it is for this reason that abnormalities in chromosome number are usually attributed to the female rather than the male gamete.

ABNORMALITIES IN CHROMOSOME NUMBER (ANEUPLOID CELLS)

The most common event producing abnormal chromosome numbers (aneuploidy) is **nondisjunction**. When nondisjunction occurs, the chromosomes are unequally distributed between the daughter cells so that one cell receives an extra chromosome (trisomy) and the other cell is missing that chromosome (monosomy). **NONDISJUNCTION CAN OCCUR ANYTIME A CELL DIVIDES (MITOTICALLY OR MEIOTICALLY) AND CAN AFFECT EITHER AUTOSOMAL OR SEX CHROMOSOMES.** It is generally accepted that one of the most frequent causes for nondisjunction is delayed or asynchronous division of centromeres during late metaphase.

MEIOTIC NONDISJUNCTION

During gametogenesis, nondisjunction results in the production of two abnormal gametes (haploid plus one or haploid minus one chromosome). If one of the abnormal gametes participates in fertilization an aneuploid zygote is produced which either possesses an extra chromosome (sex or autosomal trisomy) or lacks a chromosome (sex or autosomal monosomy). Individuals developing from these abnormal zygotes will be either trisomic or monosomic for the chromosome involved.

Zygotes with Autosomal Aneuploidy. Although 22 pairs of autosomal chromosomes are present in human zygotes and any chromosome can be affected by nondisjunction (all have been reported in aborted material), only a few (trisomic only) complete development to present as postnatal medical problems.

Autosomal Monosomy.   True monosomic conditions involving any of the 22 autosomal chromosomes have not been reported to complete intrauterine development and are generally considered to be **invariably lethal.**

Autosomal Trisomy.   Trisomic conditions for autosomal chromosomes are usually but not invariably lethal. The only common autosomal trisomic condition with long term survival is trisomy 21 (Down's syndrome). **Note:** A trisomy 22 which is similar to classical Down's has been reported with some frequency; trisomy 13 (Patau's syndrome) and trisomy 18 (Edward's syndrome) are occasionally reported but these individuals rarely survive beyond the first few months of postnatal life.

AUTOSOMAL NONDISJUNCTION

TRISOMY   MONOSOMY

The incidence of trisomy and almost all other clinical syndromes involving aneuploid gametes and zygotes (autosomal and sex chromosome aneuploidy) can be correlated with maternal age. The increased frequency of nondisjunction with advancing maternal age is usually attributed to the fact that the first meiotic division of all ova begins during fetal life. Ova produced during the later years of the reproductive life span are very old and have been subjected to the cumulative environmental (radiation, chemicals, therapeutic drugs, viral infections) and physiological (endocrine changes) effects of aging. In males, spermatogenesis occurs throughout life and the entire process from the last replication of DNA by the primary spermatocytes to the appearance of mature labeled sperm in the ejaculate is only about 64 days.

Zygotes with Sex Chromosome Aneuploidy.   In contrast to the small number of aneuploid conditions resulting from unequal distribution of the 22 pairs of autosomes, nondisjunction affecting the single pair of sex chromosomes may produce zygotes and adult individuals of at least four basic genotypes. Monosomic and trisomic conditions for sex chromosomes are well known clinically and are relatively common.

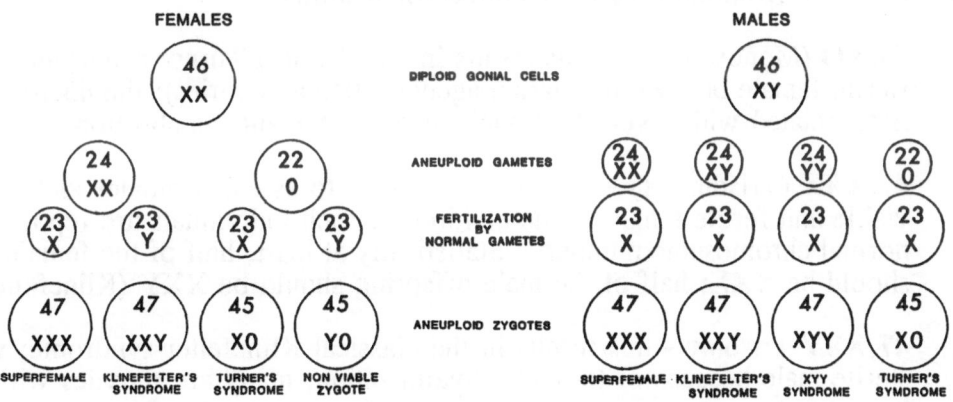

Abnormal numbers of sex chromosomes in a zygote do not appear to produce the same degree of developmental disturbances (lethality) as those produced by abnormal numbers of autosomal chromosomes. Two unusual conditions are thought to contribute to this marked reduction in lethality.

1.   The Y-chromosome of males appears to possess very few genes other than those responsible for maleness.

2.   Only one X-chromosome is required for almost normal function in diploid somatic cells; all other X-chromosomes which may be present become almost totally inactivated (nonfunctional), i.e., the **Lyon effect**. The inactivated X-chromosomes can be visualized in the nuclei of interphase cells as **sex chromatin** or **Barr bodies**.

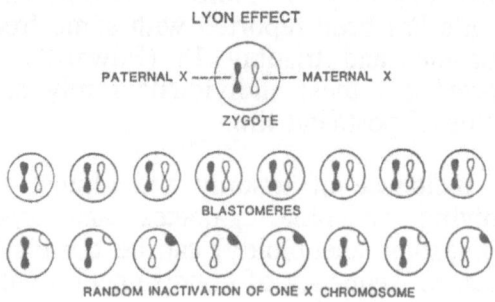

The number of Barr bodies visualized in any cell (normal or aneuploid) will always be one less than the total number of X-chromosomes present; the functional X-chromosome cannot be visualized because it is in the extended form required for transcription.

Note: The Lyon effect (X-chromosome inactivation) is initiated during the early stages of embryonic development and inactivation of the maternal or paternal X-chromosome is random (50:50). However, once the selection for inactivation of the maternal or paternal chromosome is made, all progeny of the cell will continue to inactivate the same X-chromosome. In this sense, all women are "X-chromosome mosaics" with half their somatic cells using the maternal X-chromosome and the other half using the paternal.

The abnormal sex chromosome conditions theoretically possible include both monosomic and trisomic conditions. The possibilities are summarized below.

1.   **45,YO** (Monosomy Y) - invariably lethal; no viable zygote is formed because at least one X-chromosome is required for viability.

2.   **45,XO** (Monosomy X) - this results in the classical Turner syndrome; viable but sterile female because of ovarian agenesis (streak ovaries); the 45,XO condition is associated with a very high incidence of spontaneous abortion.

3.   **47,XXX** (Trisomy X) - commonly referred to as superfemales and results in a viable and fertile female. The children of such individuals are reported to have normal chromosome numbers. Statistically at least, half of the female offspring should be XXX; half of the male offspring should be XXY (Klinefelter's).

4.   **47,XXY** Trisomy - this results in the classical Klinefelter syndrome; viable but sterile male because of testicular hyalinization; many are mosaics with multiple karyotypes.

5.   **47,XYY** Trisomy - viable and fertile male; offspring are usually reported to have normal karyotypes.

With the exception of the 45,YO condition, which produces no viable zygote, various mosaic combinations for the others are known. It is generally assumed that individuals with abnormal numbers of chromosomes develop from aneuploid zygotes formed when abnormal ova are fertilized by normal sperm, but it should be emphasized that comparable aneuploid zygotes are known to be produced when normal ova are fertilized by abnormal sperm. In both of the preceding situations, the abnormal zygote is a direct result of meiotic nondisjunction during gametogenesis. It should be noted however, that since nondisjunction can occur anytime a cell divides, abnormalities in chromosome number can also be produced at other times by mitotic nondisjunction.

MITOTIC NONDISJUNCTION

Mitotic nondisjunction during the earliest stages of embryonic development may result in aneuploid individuals with mixed populations of somatic cells, i.e., mixed karyotypes; individuals originating from mitotic nondisjunctions are referred to as **mosaics**.

When mitotic nondisjunction occurs in what was initially a normal diploid embryo, the body of the surviving mosaic individual is comprised of a mixed population of normal and abnormal (aneuploid) cells. The presence of normal cell populations in mosaics increases the chances of survival by reducing the severity of the coexisting aneuploidy, e.g., low fertility rather than complete sterility.

When mitotic nondisjunction occurs in embryos which are already aneuploid (meiotic plus mitotic nondisjunction) the somatic cells of the resulting mosaic individual is comprised entirely of abnormal aneuploid cells. The presence of two different populations appears to decrease the chances of survival by contributing to the severity of the pre-existing aneuploid condition, i.e., increasing rate of spontaneous abortion. Many 47,XXY (Klinefelter's) individuals are mosaics and may possess cell populations exhibiting two, three or more karyotypes. The prevalence of mosaicism in Klinefelter's syndrome has been attributed to a "chronically late-replicating" centromere (asynchronous division) which predisposes to repeated episodes of mitotic nondisjunction.

OTHER CAUSES FOR ABNORMAL CHROMOSOME NUMBERS

Abnormal chromosome numbers can also be produced by other less common mechanisms, i.e., anaphase lag. In anaphase lag a chromosome (autosome or sex) is actually lost from one daughter cell to produce a single abnormal monosomic cell; the other cell is normal. This condition is less serious than nondisjunction because only one-half of the cells produced are abnormal. If the loss involved an autosome, the condition would be self-limiting because of the lethality factor; if it involved the Y-chromosome it would contribute to the population of mosaic 45,XO (Turner's) individuals. Anaphase lag is also thought to involve a defective centromere.

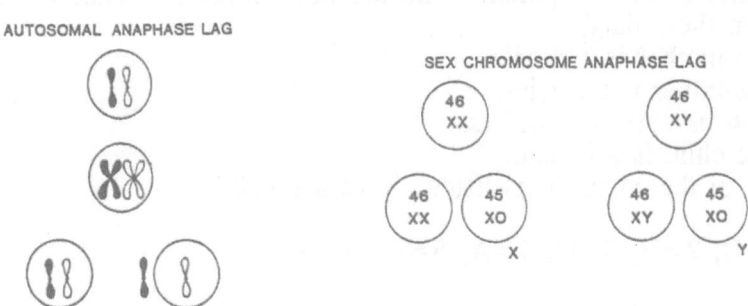

QUESTIONS: Chapter 1 - Gametogenesis

1. All of the following statements concerning chromosomes in diploid cells are true **EXCEPT**:
   A. Autosomal chromosomes are homologous in males.
   B. Autosomal chromosomes are nonhomologous in females.
   C. Sex chromosomes are homologous in females.
   D. Sex chromosomes are nonhomologous in males.
   E. The chromosome number is 46.

2. The chromatids of a partially duplicated chromosome remain joined and cannot separate as complete chromosomes until the:
   A. cytoplasm divides
   B. centromere divide
   C. centriole divides
   D. nucleolus divides
   E. nuclear membrane disappears

3. Separation of chromatids occurs during late:
   A. interphase
   B. prophase
   C. metaphase
   D. anaphase
   E. telophase

4. If the sex of a developing individual is MALE, it can be determined that an ovum:
   A. with an X-chromosome was fertilized by a Y-bearing sperm
   B. with a Y-chromosome was fertilized by a Y-bearing sperm
   C. with an X-chromosome was fertilized by an X-bearing sperm
   D. with a Y-chromosome was fertilized by an X-bearing sperm
   E. It can not be determined which combination of gametes combined to produce this individual

5. In females, the first meiotic division begins during:
   A. fetal life
   B. infancy
   C. early puberty (onset of sexual maturation)
   D. adult life immediately before ovulation
   E. adult life immediately after fertilization

6. A child with agammaglobulinemia (a sex-linked recessive disorder carried on the X-chromosome) is born to parents who are both normal. What valid conclusion can be drawn from these data?
   A. The mother is a carrier.
   B. The father is a carrier.
   C. Both parents are carriers.
   D. The child is a female.
   E. All of the conclusions listed above are valid.

Answers: 1=B, 2=B, 3=C, 4=A, 5=A, 6=A

CHAPTER 2: FEMALE REPRODUCTIVE CYCLE

Human females undergo sexual cycles which prepare the reproductive system for pregnancy; these cycles are controlled by the combined action of the hypothalamus, pituitary, ovary and uterus. The **ovarian cycle** is regulated as a direct response to pituitary gonadotropins, i.e., follicle stimulating hormone (FSH) and luteinizing hormone (LH); the **uterine cycle** is regulated as a direct response to hormones produced by the ovary (estrogen and progesterone).

The **ovarian cycle** has three major features:

1. **An initial phase of follicular development.** This occurs in response to relatively low and tonic secretion of FSH and LH by the pituitary gland. This phase culminates in increasing blood levels of estrogen produced by the maturing follicle.
2. **A midcycle surge of gonadotropins.** This phase is elicited by the rising blood levels of estrogen. The surge of gonadotropins, particularly LH, results in ovulation.
3. **A post-ovulatory phase of high circulating progesterone levels and low circulating gonadotropin levels.** Progesterone is secreted by the corpus luteum. LH promotes steroidogenesis of the corpus luteum.

The Gonadotropins are secreted by the pituitary gland. Their secretion is dependent upon gonadotropin-releasing hormone (GnRH) released by the hypothalamus into the hypothalamic-hypophyseal portal vessels. Pulsatile secretion of GnRH by the hypothalamus is responsible for the pulsatile secretion of gonadotropins by the pituitary gland. Estrogen and other factors (inhibin) released by the ovary regulate the secretion of gonadotropins by acting directly upon the pituitary gland. In addition, progesterone secreted by the corpus luteum during the post-ovulatory cycle can effect gonadotropin secretion by the pituitary gland, either by acting directly upon the pituitary gland or indirectly upon the hypothalamus.

Pituitary Follicle Stimulating Hormone (FSH) is released by the pituitary gland in a pulsatile manner and causes ovarian follicles to ripen and produce estrogen. FSH induces granulosa cells to synthesize the aromatization enzymes required to convert precursor steroids (androgens) to physiologically active estrogen. The precursor steroids (androgens including testosterone) are produced by the thecal cells in response to LH stimulation.

Estrogens produced by the ripening ovarian follicles stimulate the repair and proliferation of uterine mucosa which was lost during the preceding menstrual slough. Rising blood levels of estrogen, due almost entirely to the dominant follicle, stimulate the midcycle production of LH by the pituitary gonadotropins. An abrupt increase in estrogen blood level near the middle of the menstrual cycle is associated with the "LH surge" preceding ovulation on or about midcycle, i.e., day 14. The first meiotic division which was begun during fetal life is finally completed about the time of ovulation.

Pituitary Luteinizing Hormone (LH) converts the granulosa cells of the ruptured Graafian follicle into the progesterone-secreting **granulosa lutein cells**. LH also acts to promote steroidogenesis by the corpus luteum.

Progesterone produced by the developing corpus luteum initiates the secretory phase of the uterine mucosa (endometrium). These secretory changes in the endometrium occur while the ovum (or cleaving zygote) is traversing the uterine tube (3-4 days). The endometrium must be in the progestational or secretory phase for implantation of the blastocyst to occur. Progesterone is also important in maintaining the post-ovulatory phase of the cycle in which gonadotropin secretion is low, follicular development is held in check, and no gonadotropin surges can be elicited.

If fertilization does not occur, the corpus luteum will degenerate. The life span of the corpus luteum appears to be under the control of factors intrinsic to the ovary. The loss of the corpus luteum results in loss of circulating progesterone and the cycle begins again.

The post-ovulatory events in the reproductive cycle are relatively constant with menstruation occurring about 14 days after ovulation, i.e., on the 28th day of the menstrual cycle. Variability in cycle length whether between different individuals or between different cycles of the same individual are almost invariably due to variations in the duration of the follicular phase.

The sexual cycle is interrupted by pregnancy. The trophoblastic cells of the conceptus produce an LH-like hormone, chorionic gonadotropin, which rescues the corpus luteum from impending regression and maintains its continued function in early pregnancy. A functional corpus luteum is essential for early gestation, until the placenta can assume the endocrine activities at about 6 weeks of development.

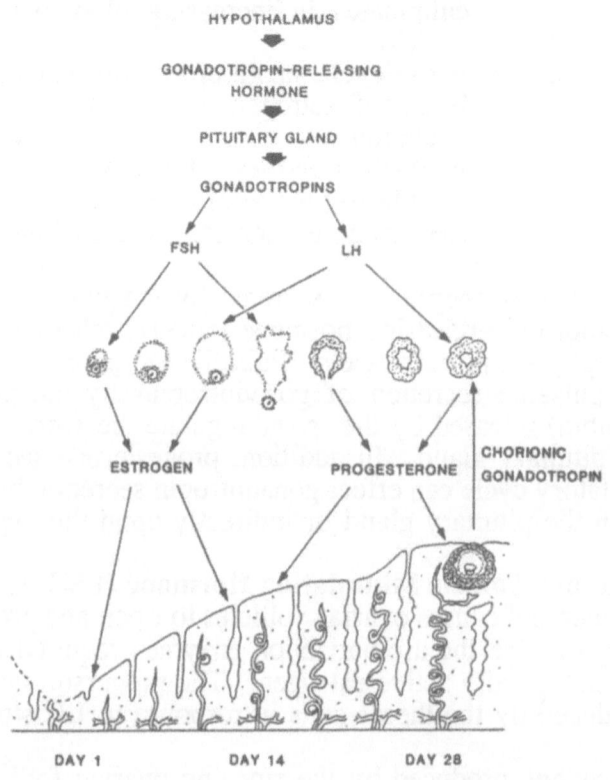

FEMALE REPRODUCTIVE SYSTEM

HYPOTHALAMUS

GONADOTROPIN-RELEASING HORMONE

PITUITARY GLAND

GONADOTROPINS

FSH   LH

ESTROGEN   PROGESTERONE   CHORIONIC GONADOTROPIN

DAY 1   DAY 14   DAY 28

QUESTIONS: Chapter 2 - Female Reproductive Cycle

1. Growth and development of ovarian follicles is a **DIRECT** response to stimulation by:
   A. gonadotropic hormones from the pituitary
   B. gonadotropin-releasing hormones
   C. progesterone from the corpus luteum
   D. chorionic gonadotropin
   E. hormones produced by the dominant follicle

2. The androgenic prohormones utilized by developing ovarian follicles for estrogen synthesis are thought to originate from the:
   A. primary oocyte
   B. granulosa cells
   C. thecal cells
   D. adrenal cortex
   E. pituitary gonadotropins

3. Induction of the aromatization enzymes required for estrogen synthesis by the ovary is attributed to an effect of:
   A. FSH on the primary oocytes
   B. LH on the primary oocytes
   C. FSH on thecal cells
   D. LH on granulosa cells
   E. FSH on granulosa cells

4. In a woman with a 35-day menstrual cycle, ovulation would be expected to occur on or about day:
   A. 7
   B. 14
   C. 21
   D. 28
   E. 35

5. The secretory phase of the uterine mucosa is a **DIRECT** response to stimulation by:
   A. progesterone
   B. estrogen
   C. human chorionic gonadotropin
   D. luteinizing hormone
   E. follicle stimulating hormone

6. During pregnancy, prolongation of the functional life span of the corpus luteum is due to:
   A. secretion of LH by the pituitary gonadotropins
   B. production of chorionic gonadotropin by the conceptus
   C. progesterone production by the placenta
   D. estrogen production by the placenta
   E. an inhibitory effect of prolactin

Answers: 1=A, 2=C, 3=E, 4=C, 5=A, 6=B

CHAPTER 3: FERTILIZATION AND PREGNANCY

FERTILIZATION

Sperm entry normally occurs shortly after ovulation (12-24 hours) and while the ovum (actually secondary oocyte) is located in the upper part of the uterine tube **(ampulla)**. Before fertilization can be effected, however, the sperm must traverse the layer of adherent granulosa cells **(corona radiata)** and **zona pellucida** surrounding the ovum. Penetration is facilitated by enzymes **(hyaluronidase** and **acrosin)** present in the acrosomal vesicle of the sperm. These enzymes are released by exocytosis of the acrosomal vesicle (acrosome reaction). After the gametes are in contact, plasma membrane fusion appears to incorporate the entire sperm (nucleus and organelles) into the cytoplasmic mass of the ovum; the second polar body is formed at this time. Formation of the second polar body indicates completion of meiosis II by the secondary oocyte; unfertilized ova do not complete meiosis II. **Triploid zygotes** containing three complete sets of chromosomes are thought to originate at the time of fertilization. (The term 'ploid' refers to complete multiples of the haploid (N) chromosome number, e.g., diploid (2N), triploid (3N), tetraploid (4N), etc.).

Explanations for the extra set of chromosomes are:

1.   simultaneous fertilization by two sperm (dispermy).
2.   failure of the oocyte to complete meiosis II with retention of the chromosome complement normally distributed to the second polar body.

Triploid zygotes are usually aborted spontaneously during early pregnancy, but a few have been reported to survive until term.

Fertilization:

1.   provides the stimulus for completion of the second meiotic division.
2.   restores the diploid number of chromosomes.
3.   determines the genetic sex of the new individual.
4.   initiates cleavage (24-30 hours post-fertilization).
5.   allows species variation by providing new combinations of genetic material.

NOTE: Fertilization provides the third mechanism for ensuring variation in the conceptus. Two earlier recombinations occurred in both parents during gametogenesis. The first recombination took place during synapsis (prophase I) when crossing-over occurred between homologous chromosomes; the second occurred with independent assortment of chromosomes during the reduction division (anaphase I).

CLEAVAGE

As the zygote passes down the uterine tube, repeated mitotic divisions **(cleavages)** produce a solid ball of cells **(morula)** consisting of about 12-16 formative cells called **blastomeres**. While the developing morula traverses the uterine tube (3-4 days), progesterone produced by the rapidly developing corpus luteum brings the endometrium into the secretory phase required for implantation.

BLASTOCYST FORMATION

After reaching the uterine cavity, the blastomeres of the morula become arranged in the form of a hollow, fluid-filled structure referred to as the **blastocyst**. Shortly after its formation, the wall of the blastocyst and a receptive endometrium will be brought into contact by disappearance of the zona pellucida. If attachment and implantation proceed, pregnancy occurs.

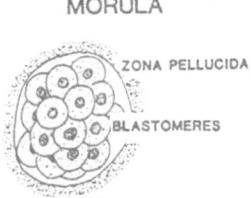

MORULA

IMPLANTATION

At the time of implantation, the blastocyst consists of an **inner cell mass** (embryoblast) which will form the embryo and an outer layer of **trophoblastic cells** which encloses the blastocyst cavity and the inner cell mass. At about 6 days, the trophoblastic cells above the inner cell mass attach to the uterine wall, penetrate the endometrial epithelium and proceed to invade the underlying stroma. Implantation is complete and the uterine mucosa is completely reepithelialized by the end of the second week, i.e., about 14 days. Some blood loss may occur during implantation and be mistaken for menstrual bleeding; this may cause erroneous calculations of expected delivery dates.

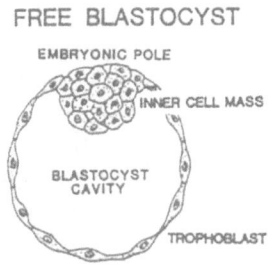

FREE BLASTOCYST

PREGNANCY

The regular sexual cycle is interrupted by the presence of an implanting blastocyst (embryo). The trophoblastic cells of the implanting blastocyst produce an LH-like hormone, **(chorionic gonadotropin)** which prevents degeneration of the corpus luteum; increasing levels of chorionic gonadotropin maintain the corpus luteum thereby assuring adequate progesterone levels for pregnancy. Almost all pregnancy tests are based on detecting the presence of chorionic gonadotropin in the maternal urine.

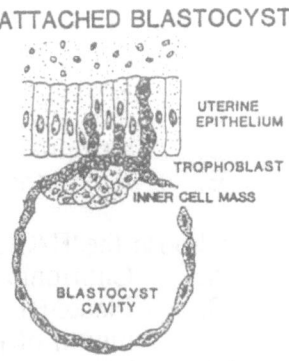

ATTACHED BLASTOCYST

DURATION OF PREGNANCY

The actual time required for human development (fertilization to parturition) is 266 days or 38 weeks. However, since the time of fertilization is usually not known, the date of the last menstrual period (LMP) is used to estimate the expected date of parturition, i.e., 280 days (266 + 14 days) or 40 weeks.

QUESTIONS: Chapter 3 - Fertilization and Pregnancy

1.   The acrosomal reaction:
      A.   releases the enzymes hyaluronidase and acrosin from the acrosomal vesicle
      B.   facilitates sperm penetration of the corona radiata
      C.   normally occurs in the ampulla of the uterine tube
      D.   facilitates sperm penetration of the zona pellucida
      E.   all of the above

2.   Fertilization normally occurs while the ovum is located in the:
      A.   posterior fornix of the vagina
      B.   uterine cavity
      C.   ampulla of the uterine tube
      D.   peritoneal cavity
      E.   antrum of the follicle

3.   Union of the male and female gametes is a process which:
      A.   induces the secondary oocyte to complete the second meiotic division
      B.   determines the sex of the zygote
      C.   restores the diploid number of chromosomes
      D.   provides for genetic variability
      E.   all of the above

4.   Which of the following is **NOT** a requirement for implantation of the blastocyst?
      A.   disappearance of the trophoblast
      B.   disappearance of the corona radiata
      C.   disappearance of the zona pellucida
      D.   attachment to the endometrium
      E.   a secretory endometrium

5.   Choose the **INCORRECT** statement.
      A.   Chorionic gonadotropin is produced within a week following implantation.
      B.   Placental progesterone is important in maintaining pregnancy after the third month of pregnancy.
      C.   The corpus luteum of pregnancy persists longer than the corpus luteum of menstruation.
      D.   The physiological effects of chorionic gonadotropin are mediated indirectly through its action on the pituitary.
      E.   The corpus luteum regresses during the last half of pregnancy.

6.   The physiological effects of chorionic gonadotropin are almost identical to those of:
      A.   estrogen
      B.   progesterone
      C.   hypothalamic releasing hormones
      D.   follicle stimulating hormone
      E.   luteinizing hormone

Answers: 1=E, 2=C, 3=E, 4=A, 5=D, 6=E

CHAPTER 4: IMPLANTATION AND FORMATION OF THE DECIDUAE

UTERINE MUCOSA

The secretory uterine mucosa consists of three well defined layers: stratum compactum, stratum spongiosum and stratum basale. The **superficial stratum (compactum)** is invaded by the implanting blastocyst and plays an active role in the implantation process. The **middle stratum (spongiosum)** contains the secretory portions of the well-developed uterine glands; during the later stages of pregnancy, when secretory activity of the glands ceases, the spongiosum cannot be visualized as a discrete and clearly defined layer. The **deepest stratum (basale)** contains the fundus of the uterine glands and does not exhibit cyclical changes during the menstrual cycle; it remains intact after the menstrual slough and after parturition to regenerate the more superficial layers.

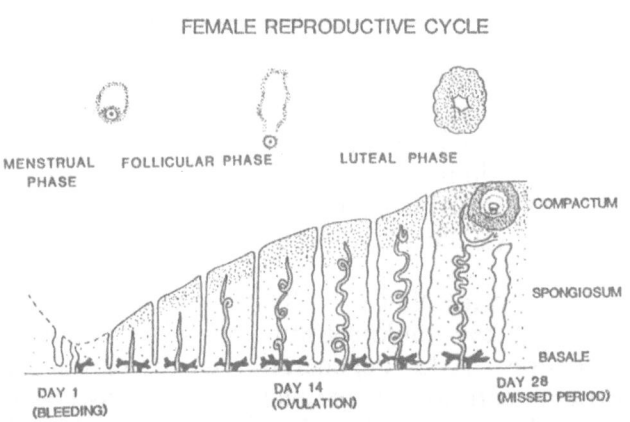

FEMALE REPRODUCTIVE CYCLE

MENSTRUAL PHASE　FOLLICULAR PHASE　LUTEAL PHASE

COMPACTUM

SPONGIOSUM

BASALE

DAY 1 (BLEEDING)　DAY 14 (OVULATION)　DAY 28 (MISSED PERIOD)

The two upper layers (compactum and spongiosum) are sometimes referred to as the **stratum functionalis** because both layers are lost and regenerated regularly during the reproductive cycles and because of their combined importance during implantation and pregnancy.

BLASTOCYST

During implantation, the trophoblastic cells forming the wall of the blastocyst differentiate into two layers. The inner layer of trophoblast is composed of discrete cells (Langhans' layer) and is referred to as the **cytotrophoblast**; the outer layer is composed of a multinucleate protoplasmic mass lacking cell boundaries and is referred to as the **syncytiotrophoblast** or syncytial layer. The syncytiotrophoblast is a **highly invasive and ingressive structure** and is responsible for the invasion of the blastocyst into the superficial stratum. As implantation proceeds, the syncytiotrophoblast becomes greatly thickened and permeated by numerous spaces or **lacunae**. As lacunar spaces form, they fill with blood originating from adjacent maternal vessels disrupted by the rapidly developing blastocyst. Eventually, the blood filled spaces will coalesce to form the intervillous vascular channels of the placenta. Growth of the syncytial layer appears to occur by recruitment or incorporation of cells derived from the cytotrophoblast. Thymidine labelling has shown that the nuclei in the syncytial layer do not incorporate thymidine unlike those of the cytotrophoblast; the labelled nuclei of the cytotrophoblast later appear within the syncytial layer.

ABNORMAL IMPLANTATION SITES

Ectopic pregnancy occurs when the blastocyst implants outside the uterus, e.g., uterine tube, peritoneal cavity, ovary. The underlying cause for implantation in these abnormal sites is usually attributed to **delayed tubal transport** of the developing conceptus. Chronic inflammation of the uterine tube with partial destruction of the tubal mucosa (endometriosis, gonorrhea, tuberculosis) is known to delay transport. Tubal pregnancies usually rupture during the second month causing severe internal hemorrhage in the mother and death of the embryo.

DECIDUAE

During pregnancy, the uterine mucosa is referred to as the **decidua** and is divided into three areas determined by their relationship to the implanted blastocyst.

Decidua Basalis.   The basalis is that portion of the endometrium located below or deep to the implanted blastocyst; it will form the **maternal portion of the placenta**.

Decidua Capsularis.   The capsularis is that portion of the endometrium covering or superficial to the implanted blastocyst; it will subsequently fuse with all of the remaining endometrium of the uterus, i.e., parietalis, to obliterate the uterine cavity. After fusion, the capsularis degenerates (about 22 weeks).

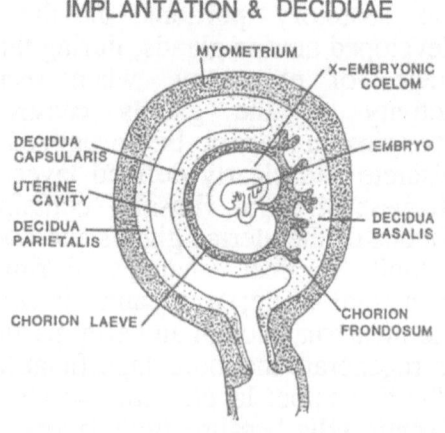

IMPLANTATION & DECIDUAE

Decidua Parietalis.   The parietalis includes all portions of the endometrium other than the site of implantation. After degeneration of the capsularis (and superficial part of the parietalis), the deeper parietalis fuses with the nonplacental portion of the chorion (chorion laeve); this fusion facilitates amniotic fluid exchange across the thin juxtaposed walls of the amnion and chorion laeve.

After parturition, the deciduae are shed as part of the afterbirth; the superficial or functional layers of the endometrium (compactum and spongiosum) regenerate from the persisting stratum basale. **(Do not confuse the decidua basalis with the stratum basale).**

EXTRAEMBRYONIC MEMBRANES

The fetal membranes are temporary structures necessary for embryonic development; they are lost as part of the afterbirth at the time of parturition. They are referred to as the extraembryonic membranes. The extraembryonic structures appear very early and become functional (partially at least) before the developing embryo can be recognized as anything more than a double layer of epithelial cells. The four extraembryonic membranes are the: **chorion, amnion, yolk sac and allantois**. The chorion is the first to appear; its future epithelial layer is recognizable as the trophoblastic cells forming the wall of the blastocyst. After its mesenchymal and vascular components appear, the chorion will form the **fetal portion of the placenta**.

QUESTIONS: Chapter 4 - Implantation and Formation of the Deciduae

1. The most active role in the implantation process appears to be performed by:
    A. decidual cells
    B. syncytiotrophoblastic cells
    C. cytotrophoblastic cells
    D. cells of the embryoblast (inner cell mass)
    E. Langhans' cells

2. Maternal contributions to the placenta originate from the:
    A. decidua parietalis
    B. decidua capsularis
    C. decidua basalis
    D. chorion frondosum (villous chorion)
    E. chorion laeve (smooth chorion)

3. Tubal implantation is usually attributed to:
    A. delayed ovulation
    B. delayed fertilization
    C. delayed transport
    D. early implantation
    E. late implantation

4. The first extraembryonic membrane to appear during human development is the:
    A. chorion
    B. amnion
    C. allantois
    D. yolk sac
    E. umbilical cord

5. When implantation is complete, the blastocyst is located within the:
    A. stratum compactum
    B. stratum spongiosum
    C. stratum basale
    D. decidua capsularis
    E. decidua basalis

6. Which of the following does **NOT** become part of the afterbirth?
    A. decidua basalis
    B. chorion
    C. decidua parietalis
    D. stratum basale
    E. umbilical cord

7. The blastocyst most frequently implants:
    A. near the midline
    B. on the posterior uterine wall
    C. between the openings of the uterine glands
    D. with the inner cell mass directed toward the uterine mucosa
    E. all of the above

Answers: 1=B, 2=C, 3=C, 4=A, 5=A, 6=D, 7=E

CHAPTER 5: FORMATION OF THE PLACENTA

CHORIONIC CONTRIBUTIONS

Fetal Placenta.   As the lacunar spaces within the thickened syncytiotrophoblast coalesce and increase in size, irregular strands of syncytium are produced which project into the rapidly developing vascular channels. Almost immediately after their formation, cytotrophoblastic cells grow into these syncytial strands to produce the **primary** chorionic villi which are composed of trophoblastic cells only, i.e., centrally located cytotrophoblastic cells ensheathed by a layer of syncytial cells. Primary villi are converted to **secondary** chorionic villi by the invasion of a mesenchymal core derived from the extraembryonic chorionic mesoderm; vascularization of the mesenchymal core produces the functional **tertiary** chorionic villus. Initially, the entire chorionic surface is covered with villi but those adjacent to the decidua capsularis degenerate to produce the smooth (nonvillous) **chorion laeve**. Villi adjacent to the decidua basalis persist and increase in size to produce the **chorion frondosum** which becomes the fetal portion of the placenta.

DECIDUAL CONTRIBUTIONS

Maternal Placenta.   During implantation, maternal tissues and capillaries of the decidua basalis are disrupted by the invasive action of the blastocyst and as a consequence, the chorion is soon surrounded by a stagnant pool of extravasated maternal blood, tissue debris and secretions from disrupted uterine glands, i.e., **embryotroph**. Substances diffusing from the embryotroph are thought to serve as a source of nourishment for the conceptus until placental circulation begins. As development continues, larger uterine vessels (arterial and venous) are disrupted and brought into communication with the lacunar spaces. With the establishment of arterial and venous connections, maternal blood begins to circulate through the developing intervillous spaces of the chorion frondosum. While these vascular changes are taking place, cytotrophoblastic cells in the chorionic villi penetrate the ensheathing layer of syncytial cells and spread along the surface of adjacent maternal tissues to form the **cytotrophoblastic shell**. When the cytotrophoblastic shell is complete, it encloses the entire conceptus including the chorionic villi and serves as the only physical attachment between maternal tissues and those of the conceptus. The shell is interrupted only at the sites where maternal blood vessels communicate with the intervillous spaces of the fetal placenta. Chorionic villi which are attached directly to the cytotrophoblastic shell are called **anchoring villi**; free or unattached **branch villi** extend from the surfaces of anchoring villi and exhibit elaborate branching patterns within the blood filled intervillous spaces. Most of the surface area available for metabolic exchange is provided by the branch villi. The placenta is fully formed and mature by the fourth month of development.

When mature, the placenta has the following characteristics:

1.   diameter of 15-20 cm.
2.   total volume of approximately 500 ml.
3.   maternal blood volume of approximately 150 ml.
4.   maternal blood flow of approximately 600 ml/min.
5.   weight of 500-600 grams (approximately one-sixth of the fetal weight).

PLACENTAL CIRCULATION

Deoxygenated fetal blood leaves the fetus via the umbilical arteries and passes into the capillaries in the chorionic villi where gaseous and nutrient exchange occurs. Oxygenated blood returns to the fetus via the umbilical veins. A simple circulatory system (ebb and flow) is found in the embryo, yolk sac, connecting body stalk and chorion at about 21 days; by 28 days, the circulation is regular and unidirectional in all three vascular circuits, i.e., embryonic, vitelline (yolk sac) and placental (chorionic).

PLACENTAL MEMBRANE

Originally, the membrane separating the fetal and maternal blood consists of four layers:

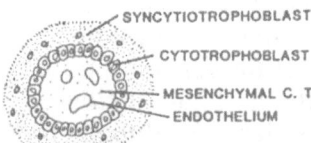

1.   syncytiotrophoblast.
2.   cytotrophoblast (Langhan's layer).
3.   mesenchymal connective tissue of the villus core.
4.   endothelium of the fetal capillaries.

Disappearance of the cytotrophoblast (Langhan's cells) as a complete layer after the fourth month and thinning of the mesenchymal layer brings the fetal capillaries into apposition with the syncytial layer during late pregnancy. Close apposition and thinning of the syncytium increases the efficiency of exchange to meet the increasing metabolic demands of the rapidly maturing fetus.

PLACENTAL FUNCTIONS

METABOLIC TRANSPORT

Nutrients.   Water, electrolytes, gases, glucose, amino acids and fatty acids cross the placental barrier readily in both directions by simple diffusion. Some active transport may be required for glucose because it is the major energy source for the fetus. Glucose levels of the fetus are normally 20-30 percent lower than those of the mother. Neutral lipids of maternal origin are thought to cross by pinocytotic activity.

Metabolites.   Urea, creatinine and creatine cross the placental barrier by simple diffusion.

ENDOCRINE FUNCTIONS

Protein Hormones.   Protein and glycoprotein hormones do not cross the placental barrier readily. Thyroxine and insulin have been reported to cross slowly but in physiologically significant amounts. Chorionic gonadotropin produced by the syncytiotrophoblast appears in maternal urine during the second week (during implantation) and is present in large amounts until the fourth month of pregnancy.

Steroid Hormones.   Steroid hormones pass the placental barrier readily unless conjugated; conjugated steroids do not cross. Progesterone is produced throughout pregnancy from precursors of maternal origin; estrogens are synthesized from precursors supplied by the fetal liver and adrenal cortex. Fetal levels of estrogen and progesterone increase throughout pregnancy and at birth, fetal levels are higher than those of the mother.

IMMUNOLOGICAL FUNCTIONS

Antibodies.   IgG antibodies are actively transferred across the placental barrier; newborn infants have passive humoral immunity acquired from the mother by selective transfer of IgG. IgA and IgM antibodies do not cross the placental barrier.   Failure of ABO blood group isoagglutinins (IgM) to cross the placental barrier explains why differences in maternal and fetal ABO blood groups rarely result in hemolytic disease of the newborn.   Hemolytic disease of the newborn (erythroblastosis fetalis) is seen most frequently when the mother is Rh negative and the fetus is Rh positive.   If the mother becomes sensitized to the Rh positive fetal cells, she responds by producing anti-Rh antibodies of the IgG type which are then transferred across the placental barrier with subsequent hemolysis of the fetal red blood cells.

INFECTIOUS AGENTS

Infectious agents of various types, e.g., viruses (rubella, HIV, cytomegalovirus), bacteria (tuberculosis, syphilis) and protozoa (toxoplasma) are known to cross the placental barrier and infect the fetus in utero. Some of the infectious agents listed above are known to be associated with a high incidence of severe congenital malformations (cytomegalovirus, rubella, toxoplasma). Rubella provides the classical example. Approximately 25 percent of infants born to mothers having rubella during the first trimester exhibit the rubella triad of: congenital cataracts, cardiac defects and deafness. Other infants infected in utero may appear normal at birth, but are nevertheless infected and may be a source of new infections among family members and/or hospital personnel - especially when unexpected.

CHEMICALS

Therapeutic Drugs.   Many drugs and chemicals cross the placental barrier readily without affecting the conceptus adversely, but some commonly used therapeutic agents, e.g., anticoagulants (warfarin), anticonvulsants (dilantin) and antitumor agents (aminopterin) are known to produce severe congenital malformations. As a general rule, the most devastating effects are produced if the teratogenic agents are administered during the embryonic or organogenesis period; thalidomide with its distinctive limb defects is a classic example. Characteristic but less severe developmental abnormalities are associated with the administration of synthetic steroids and tetracycline during pregnancy. Synthetic steroids which are potentially androgenic may masculinize the external genitalia of the female fetus resulting in ambiguous genitalia at birth.   The deciduous teeth of children whose mothers received tetracycline treatment during pregnancy are discolored and hypoplastic because this antibiotic is deposited during active mineralization (deciduous teeth mineralize before birth). Tetracycline administered during infancy and early childhood exhibit comparable defects in the permanent teeth which are formed and mineralized postnatally.

Social Drugs.   Alcohol, among the social drugs, has recently been recognized as a potent teratogen; chronic alcoholism in mothers is currently believed to be the leading cause for mental retardation.

QUESTIONS: Chapter 5 - Formation of the Placenta

1. The walls of the intervillous spaces in the placenta are lined by:
   A. maternal endothelial cells
   B. fetal endothelial cells
   C. syncytiotrophoblastic cells
   D. stromal cells of the uterine mucosa
   E. none of the above

2. The fetal membrane most intimately concerned with formation of the placenta is the:
   A. chorion
   B. amnion
   C. yolk sac
   D. allantois
   E. none of the above

3. During late pregnancy, exchange across the placental membrane is facilitated by:
   A. regression of the cytotrophoblast
   B. thinning of the syncytiotrophoblast
   C. reduction in thickness of the perivascular mesenchymal connective tissue
   D. apposition of fetal capillaries and syncytiotrophoblast
   E. all of the above

4. The following cross the placental membrane readily in both directions **EXCEPT**:
   A. free fatty acids
   B. conjugated steroids
   C. amino acids
   D. carbon dioxide
   E. creatinine

5. Which of the following structures plays an important role in attaching the conceptus to maternal tissues?
   A. cytotrophoblastic shell
   B. secondary villi
   C. intervillous spaces
   D. amnion
   E. chorion leave

6. Choose the **INCORRECT** statement concerning hemolytic disease of the newborn.
   A. Rh antibodies are transported across the placental membrane.
   B. The Rh antibodies are produced by the fetus
   C. The blood type of the mother is Rh negative.
   D. The blood type of the father is Rh positive.
   E. The blood type of the fetus is Rh positive.

7. Maternal and fetal blood mix freely in the:
   A. chorionic blood vessels
   B. intervillous spaces in the placenta
   C. maternal blood vessels
   D. amniotic cavity
   E. none of the above

Answers: 1=C, 2=A, 3=E, 4=B, 5=A, 6=B, 7=E

CHAPTER 6: FETAL MEMBRANES AND UMBILICAL CORD

CHORION

The multifunctional roles of the chorion to the implantation process and to the formation and function of the placenta have been discussed previously.

AMNION

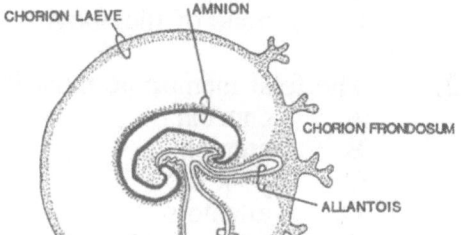

EXTRAEMBRYONIC FETAL MEMBRANES

Growth of the fetus and surrounding amniotic sac gradually obliterates the extraembryonic coelomic space and brings the membranes of the amnion and chorion into direct apposition. Obliteration of the extraembryonic coelom and apposition of the amniotic and chorionic membranes facilitates the exchange of substances between amniotic fluid and maternal blood. As growth and enlargement continue, the body stalk and yolk stalk become surrounded and ensheathed by part of the amniotic membrane which will subsequently form the external covering of the umbilical cord.

Amniotic Fluid. The source of amniotic fluid during early development is uncertain; some may be secreted by amniotic cells themselves but most of its volume appears to be absorbed or accumulated from maternal blood. During later development, the fetus contributes to the volume by excreting approximately 500 ml of urine daily; subsequent ingestion by the fetus followed by intestinal absorption and elimination via the placenta prevents excessive accumulations. At term the volume of amniotic fluid is approximately 1000 ml. Isotope studies indicate that the aqueous component is exchanged every three hours and that most of the water exchange occurs in the area where the juxtaposed membranes of the amnion and chorion laeve are fused with the decidua parietalis; somewhat smaller amounts of exchange occur in the area of the placenta proper, i.e., between the juxtaposed membranes of the amnion and chorion frondosum and decidua basalis. Renal agenesis and urethral obstruction are associated with abnormally small amount of amniotic fluid (oligohydramnios); abnormally large amounts (polyhydramnios) may occur when fetal ingestion is decreased, e.g., anencephaly (absence of a swallowing reflex) or with high intestinal obstruction (esophageal, pyloric or duodenal atresia). The amnion is lost at parturition as part of the afterbirth.

YOLK SAC

The yolk sac is nonfunctional as far as stored nutrients are concerned, but it is thought to have some role in the transfer of nutrients from the embryotroph to the embryo before placental circulation is established. It is especially important during early development because of its contributions (roof part only) to the digestive system, its role in hematopoietic functions and as the source of primitive germ cells for the next generation. By the fifth week of development the yolk sac is located within the developing umbilical cord lodged between the body stalk and ensheathing layer of the amniotic membrane. The yolk sac itself is located near the attachment of the cord to the placenta and it remains at this site throughout development. The lumen of the yolk stalk (vitelline duct) is usually obliterated and detached from the gut by the end of the embryonic period, i.e., 56 days. The yolk sac and remnants of the stalk are lost with the placenta and cord at the time of parturition.

Developmental Defects.   Failure of the yolk stalk lumen to obliterate and detach results in the production of an ileo-umbilical fistula (persistent vitelline duct) which permits intestinal contents to escape via the umbilicus when the cord is severed at parturition.   Complete or partial luminal obliteration without detachment from the gut produces, respectively, a fibrous or a cystic (vitelline cysts) cord extending from the ileum to the anterior body wall (umbilicus). Fibrous connections between the gut and body wall predispose the gut to obstruction and/or strangulation (volvulus).   In about 2% of the adult population, the proximal part of the yolk stalk persists to form a Meckel's diverticulum; these diverticula are always located on the antimesenteric side of the ileum near its termination in the caecum.   Although Meckel's diverticula are usually asymptomatic, they often contain heterotopic tissue (gastric and pancreatic) which is predisposed to inflammation, bleeding and ulceration and may progress to perforation.

ALLANTOIS

In humans, the allantois is very small (microscopic) and appears to be a rudimentary structure. Despite is microscopic size and rudimentary appearance, the allantois is essential for development to continue because its presence is required to initiate vascularization of the chorion (fetal placenta).

Note: Experimental and other evidence indicates that endodermal cells must be present to initiate blood vessel formation (angiogenesis) and the production of blood cells (hematocytopoiesis) and it is probably for this reason that angiogenesis and hematopoiesis are first seen in the splanchnic mesoderm of the yolk sac and allantois.   The somatic mesoderm of the amnion and chorion is intrinsically avascular.   The chorion becomes vascularized indirectly by vessels derived from sites of angiogenesis initiated in the splanchnic mesoderm of the body stalk by the allantoic endoderm.   Although the amnion possesses a comparable layer of somatic mesoderm, it remains almost totally avascular throughout development.

The endodermal epithelium of the allantoic diverticulum originates from the most caudal limit of the yolk sac roof and grows into the adjacent body stalk mesoderm.   Almost immediately, the allantoic vessels (umbilical, placental) differentiate and grow distally to vascularize the chorionic mesoderm.   A short time later, the allantoic region of the yolk sac roof will be incorporated into the body of the embryo to form the ventral wall or floor of the hind gut.   The proximal or embryonic portion of the allantois is referred to as the **urachus**.   Much later in development, when the hind gut becomes divided into dorsal (rectal) and ventral (urogenital) areas, the embryonic or urachal portion of the allantois retains its ventral attachment to the urogenital sinus (bladder portion) and extends cranially to the umbilicus.   Eventually, the urachus looses its lumen and becomes converted into a fibrous, cord-like structure which persists in the adult as the **median umbilical ligament**.   After birth, the umbilical arteries (allantoic) accompanying the urachus become nonfunctional, undergo fibrosis and persist in the adult as the **medial umbilical ligaments**.   The extraembryonic portions of the allantoic lumen and epithelium within the body stalk (now forming the core of the umbilical cord) degenerate. In histological preparations of the term cord, epithelial remanents of the allantoic epithelium can often be visualized between the umbilical arteries.   All extraembryonic portions of the allantois are lost with the umbilical cord and placenta at birth.

Developmental Defects.   Persistence of the urachal lumen throughout its entire length (urachal fistula) allows urine to escape vial the umbilicus when the cord is severed at birth; persistence of parts of the urachal lumen may produce cystic inclusions (urachal cysts) in the median umbilical ligament.

UMBILICAL CORD

The umbilical cord is not one of the fetal membranes. It is a composite structure formed by contributions from the:

1. connecting or body stalk which contains the allantoic epithelium and the allantoic (umbilical) arteries and vein.
2. extraembryonic portion of the yolk stalk.
3. portions of the amnion ensheathing both of the above structures.

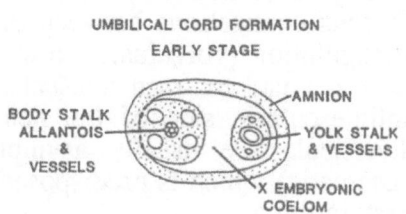

UMBILICAL CORD FORMATION
EARLY STAGE

BODY STALK
ALLANTOIS
&
VESSELS

AMNION
YOLK STALK
& VESSELS
X EMBRYONIC
COELOM

Subsequent fusion of these three components obliterates the extraembryonic coelomic space (umbilical coelom) to produce the definitive umbilical cord. During later stages of development, the right umbilical (allantois) vein disappears so that the normal cord has two arteries and one vein. At term, the umbilical cord is 1-2 cm in diameter and 50-55 cm in length; the minimum length for successful delivery is approximately 30 cm. The umbilical cord is lost with the placenta at birth.

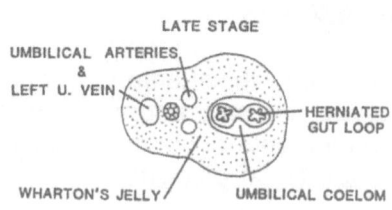

LATE STAGE

UMBILICAL ARTERIES
&
LEFT U. VEIN

HERNIATED
GUT LOOP

WHARTON'S JELLY
UMBILICAL COELOM

Developmental Defects. True knots are sometimes found in the normal cord and may compromise the fetal blood supply when the cord is subjected to tension; exceptionally long cords predispose to knot formation. The attachment site of the umbilical cord is determined by the orientation of the blastocyst at implantation. If the embryonic pole attaches first (normal position), the cord is attached centrally. If the blastocyst attaches to one side of the embryonic pole (abnormal position), the cord is attached to the placental margin. Persistence of the extraembryonic coelom near the attachment of the umbilicus to the fetus may contribute or predispose to some types of umbilical hernia.

QUESTIONS: Chapter 6 - Fetal Membranes and Umbilical Cord

1. During early development, the extraembryonic coelomic space is gradually obliterated by expansion or growth of the:
   A. amniotic sac
   B. yolk sac
   C. chorion laeve
   D. chorion frondosum
   E. extraembryonic mesoderm

2. Extraembryonic structures which are known to possess important hematopoietic functions during early embryonic development include the:
   A. yolk sac and chorion
   B. chorion and amnion
   C. amnion and allantois
   D. allantois and yolk sac
   E. none of the above combinations is correct

3. The placental or umbilical vessels are usually considered to originate from the vasculature associated with the:
   A. allantois and body stalk
   B. yolk sac and yolk stalk
   C. amnion
   D. chorion laeve
   E. none of the above

4. During the last half of fetal life, which of the following extraembryonic structures must be traversed by water molecules to effect nonplacental amniotic fluid exchange?
   A. amnion and extraembryonic coelom
   B. amnion, extraembryonic coelom and chorion frondosum
   C. extraembryonic coelom and chorion frondosum
   D. amnion and chorion laeve
   E. extraembryonic coelom only

5. Which of the following are normally lost or disappear at some stage of human development (early or late)?
   A. decidua capsularis
   B. extraembryonic coelom
   C. umbilical coelom
   D. uterine cavity
   E. all of the above

6. The primitive germ cells of the developing embryo are believed to originate from the:
   A. yolk sac
   B. germinal epithelium
   C. primitive streak
   D. body stalk
   E. none of the above

Answers: 1=A; 2=D; 3=A; 4=D; 5=E; 6=A

CHAPTER 7: EARLY DEVELOPMENT OF THE CONCEPTUS

FORMATION OF THE BILAMINAR EMBRYO

Before implantation of the blastocyst is complete, a small, fluid-filled space appears within the cluster of blastomeres forming the inner cell mass (embryoblast); this space is the **amniotic cavity**. As the amniotic cavity enlarges, the remaining blastomeres of the inner cell mass become rearranged to form a flattened disk consisting of two layers of simple epithelium arranged back-to-back; this structure is the **bilaminar embryo**. Differentiation of the embryonic disk allows the developing conceptus to be divided into **embryonic** and **extraembryonic areas**; subsequent developmental changes will continue to accentuate the boundaries between embryonic and extraembryonic regions of the conceptus.

Epiblast. The cells covering the floor of the amniotic cavity (upper surface of the embryonic disk) are columnar in shape and are referred to as the **epiblast** (ectoderm). At the peripheral edge of the embryonic disk, the epiblast is continuous with the amniotic epithelium (extraembryonic ectoderm) forming the dome or roof of the amniotic cavity.

Hypoblast. The blastomeres forming the deeper epithelial layer are cuboidal in shape and are referred to as the **hypoblast** (visceral endoderm). The visceral endodermal cells extend beyond the bilaminar disk and are continuous with the parietal endoderm lining the primary yolk sac (previously referred to as the exocoelomic membrane).

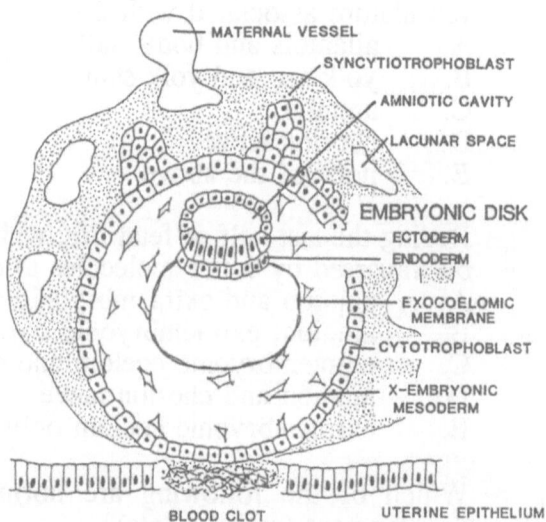

BILAMINAR EMBRYONIC DISK

- MATERNAL VESSEL
- SYNCYTIOTROPHOBLAST
- AMNIOTIC CAVITY
- LACUNAR SPACE

EMBRYONIC DISK
- ECTODERM
- ENDODERM

- EXOCOELOMIC MEMBRANE
- CYTOTROPHOBLAST
- X-EMBRYONIC MESODERM

BLOOD CLOT   UTERINE EPITHELIUM

Note: During subsequent stages of development, the supporting (connective) tissues for the epithelial layers of the conceptus (embryonic and extraembryonic) are derived from some type of mesoderm. The supporting tissues for the epithelial components of the extraembryonic membranes, i.e., ectoderm of the amnion and chorion (trophoblast) and the endoderm of the yolk sac and allantois, are derived from extraembryonic mesoderm; the supporting tissues for the ectoderm and endoderm of the embryo proper develop from embryonic mesoderm.

EXTRAEMBRYONIC MESODERM FORMATION

It should be noted that the extraembryonic mesoderm of the fetal membranes (chorion, amnion, yolk sac, allantois) appears earlier and originates from a source different than that of the embryonic mesoderm. Extraembryonic mesoderm is required very early to prepare **in advance** the vascular elements (vessels and blood cells) which will soon be needed to complete a functional (oxygen transporting) placental circulation for the embryo. Primitive red blood cells with hemoglobin can be identified easily in the yolk sac mesoderm on the eighteenth day of development; a rudimentary 'ebb and flow' circulation begins two or three days later. After this time (about 21 days), growth of the embryo is described as being 'almost explosive'.

The cells comprising the extraembryonic mesoderm were previously believed to be derived from the inner layer of the blastocyst wall (cytotrophoblast). The most recent evidence, however, suggests that the extraembryonic mesoderm is derived from parietal endodermal cells (exocoelomic membrane) lining the primary yolk sac. Extraembryonic mesodermal cells proliferate until almost all of the blastocyst cavity is occupied by a loose network of mesodermal cells (mesenchyme) separated by large amounts of extracellular matrix.

EXTRAEMBRYONIC COELOM FORMATION

While the extraembryonic portion of the yolk sac is being completed, isolated spaces begin to appear within the extraembryonic mesoderm filling the blastocyst (chorionic) cavity. These spaces enlarge rapidly and eventually coalesce to form a single, large **extraembryonic coelom**.

Except in the most caudal area of the embryonic disk, extension of the extraembryonic coelom separates the amnion, yolk sac and remaining portion of the embryonic disk from the blastocyst wall. The persisting strip of extraembryonic mesoderm is the **body stalk** and it is the only direct connection remaining between the embryo and the developing fetal placenta (chorion frondosum). A short time later, a small diverticulum (allantois) originating from the caudal limits of the yolk sac roof will grow into the body stalk mesoderm and initiate the formation of the allantoic (umbilical, placental) blood vessels. The persisting connection between the body stalk and chorion allows the allantois vessels to reach and vascularize the chorion (fetal placenta).

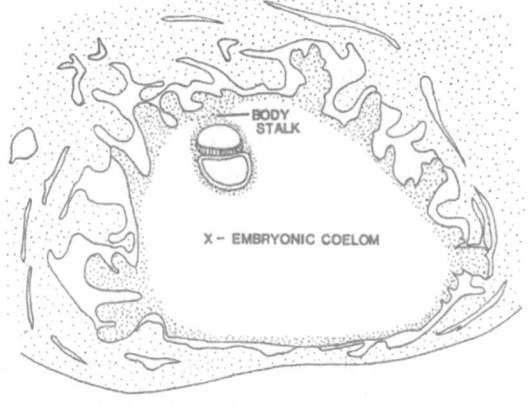

BILAMINAR EMBRYO
EXTRAEMBRYONIC MESODERM & COELOM FORMATION

Formation of the extraembryonic coelom divides the extraembryonic mesoderm into two layers which are referred to as the **somatic** and **splanchnic** layers of the extraembryonic mesoderm. **Extraembryonic somatic mesoderm** is adjacent to the epithelium of the amnion and chorion (trophoblast); the combined layers of somatic mesoderm and epithelium form the extraembryonic somatopleura. **Extraembryonic splanchnic mesoderm** is adjacent to the endodermal epithelium of the yolk sac and allantois; the combined layers of splanchnic mesoderm and endoderm form the extraembryonic splanchnopleura.

While all of the changes described above are taking place, the bilaminar embryo has remained almost unchanged. The embryonic mesoderm is formed later and is derived from a different source than the precociously formed extraembryonic mesoderm of the fetal membranes.

FORMATION OF THE TRILAMINAR EMBRYO

Just prior to the appearance of the embryonic mesoderm, the developing embryo consists of a circular or oval shaped disk composed of:

1. **epiblast** covering the upper surface of the embryo and forming the floor of the amniotic cavity.
2. **visceral endoderm** (hypoblast) covering the lower surface of the embryo and forming the roof of the yolk sac.

At about 14 days, a groove and slight thickening appear in the ectoderm covering the upper surface of the embryonic disk; this structure is the **primitive streak** and its appearance indicates the onset of embryonic mesoderm formation and the formation of the **trilaminar embryo.** Its location toward one edge of the embryonic disk (caudal) determines the future body axes of the embryo, i.e., craniocaudal orientation and right and left sides. A slight elevation at its cranial end, **Hensen's node,** is thought to correspond to the dorsal lip of the blastopore in lower vertebrates. The primitive streak and node are usually considered to function as the primary organizer for embryonic development. The role of primary organizer has also been attributed to the prochordal plate and/or notochord.

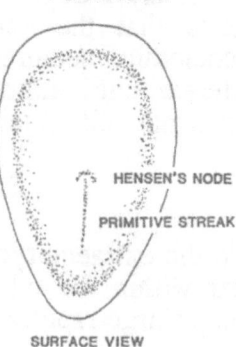

PRIMITIVE STREAK FORMATION

HENSEN'S NODE
PRIMITIVE STREAK

SURFACE VIEW

EMBRYONIC MESODERM FORMATION

Mesodermal cells proliferating from both sides of the primitive streak spread distally between the ectodermal and endodermal epithelial layers of the embryonic disk to form the third layer of the trilaminar embryonic plate. The sheets of embryonic mesoderm spread peripherally around the circumference of the embryonic disk to become continuous with the extraembryonic mesoderm of the amnion and yolk sac which had been formed earlier.

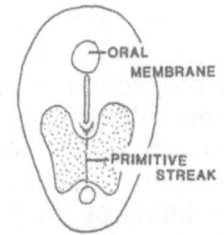

EMBRYONIC MESODERM FORMATION

ORAL MEMBRANE

PRIMITIVE STREAK

Although the sheets of embryonic mesoderm on the right and left sides do not fuse across the midline in the areas occupied by the oropharyngeal membrane, notochord, primitive streak and cloacal membrane at this time, they do invade the midline cranial to the oropharyngeal membrane to form the mesoderm for the **cardiogenic area** (heart and pericardial cavity) and the primitive body wall **above** the umbilicus. Some time later, a comparable fusion will occur across the midline caudal to the cloacal membrane to produce the mesodermal components of the primitive body wall **below** the umbilicus.

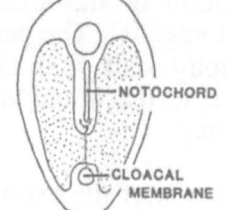

NOTOCHORD

CLOACAL MEMBRANE

Early Developmental Defects. Failure of the embryonic mesoderm to fuse across the midline **cranial** to the oropharyngeal membrane (cardiogenic area) results in heart and upper body wall defects so severe that development usually ceases. Failure of the embryonic mesoderm to fuse across the midline **caudal** to the cloacal membrane is thought to cause or be a major contributing factor to severe developmental defects involving the body wall below the umbilicus including the pubic symphysis and urethra, e.g., complete exstrophy of the urinary bladder.

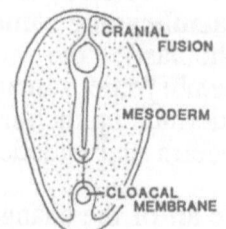

CRANIAL FUSION

MESODERM

CLOACAL MEMBRANE

EMBRYONIC ECTODERM FORMATION

The epiblast cells that remain on the surface of the embryo after gastrulation will form the ectodermal germ layer. The ectoderm will form the epithelium covering the external surface of the body, i.e., epidermis of the skin, and all parts of the nervous system.

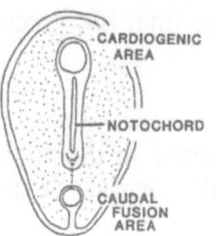

CARDIOGENIC AREA

NOTOCHORD

CAUDAL FUSION AREA

EMBRYONIC ENDODERM FORMATION

In humans it is still unclear which cell type will give rise to the endodermal germ layer. The visceral endodermal cells (hypoblast) forming the lower layer of the bilaminar disk may persist to form the endoderm. Alternatively, some of the mesenchymal cells which migrate through the primitive streak may displace the hypoblast, replacing this layer with epiblast-derived cells. In either case, the cells which comprise the endodermal germ layer will form the epithelium covering the internal surface of the body, i.e., lumen of the gut, and all of its derivatives including the respiratory system.

EMBRYONIC COELOM FORMATION

After mesoderm formation is well advanced, small, isolated spaces appear within the rapidly expanding sheets of embryonic mesoderm; extension and coalescence of the isolated spaces produce the pleural and peritoneal portions of the **embryonic coelom**. Subsequent fusion of the embryonic mesoderm cranially allows the embryonic coelom to extend across the midline to form the future **pericardial cavity**. At this time, the complete embryonic coelom has the shape of an inverted "U". Eventually, peripheral extensions bring the embryonic and extraembryonic coelomic spaces into broad communication laterally. Note that the embryonic and extraembryonic coelomic spaces remain separated in the cardiogenic or cranial area. The persisting band of mesoderm separating the two coelomic spaces in the cardiogenic area is the **septum transversum**. The septum transversum is an important land mark and will be used as a reference point throughout this book. Because it will ultimately contribute to the formation of the diaphragm, it provides a useful boundary for dividing the body into cranial and caudal halves.

Formation of the embryonic coelom divides the embryonic mesoderm into somatic and splanchnic layers which are adjacent to the ectodermal and endodermal epithelium of the embryo. The combined outer layers (ectoderm and somatic mesoderm) form the **embryonic somatopleura** or **primitive body wall**; the combined inner layers (endoderm and splanchnic mesoderm) form the **embryonic splanchnopleura** or **primitive gut wall**. Peripherally, the:

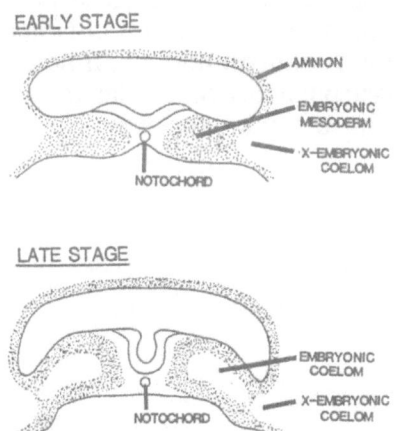

TRILAMINAR EMBRYONIC PLATE

EARLY STAGE

LATE STAGE

1. **embryonic somatopleura** or primitive body wall is continuous with the extraembryonic somatopleura of the amnion.
2. **embryonic splanchnopleura** or primitive gut wall is continuous with the extraembryonic splanchnopleura of the yolk sac.

Note: The formation of embryonic and extraembryonic 'pleura' must occur if development is to continue because the layers of ectodermal and endodermal epithelium are avascular. Even in the adult, epithelial cells are maintained by blood vessels located in the underlying connective tissue. The somatic and splanchnic layers of mesoderm are developing connective tissues for the adjacent epithelial cells; vascularization occurs almost immediately after their formation. The ectodermal and endodermal epithelia forming the oropharyngeal and cloacal membranes are firmly adherent and are, therefore, not invaded by embryonic mesoderm. As a consequence, these epithelial membranes remain avascular and subsequently degenerate to produce the oral and anal opening for the digestive tract. Occasionally, the cloacal membrane is invaded by mesoderm which then becomes vascularized and allows the membrane to persist. The developmental defect produced by a persistent cloacal membrane is **imperforate anus.**

PRIMITIVE STREAK

Mesodermal proliferation from the primitive streak continues for about two weeks; after this time, its relative size decreases and normally, it disappears without a trace. Occasionally, remnants are thought to persist in the sacrococcygeal region and give rise to tumors composed of multiple tissue types, i.e., **teratomas.** These tumors may be present at birth and may be quite large.

NOTOCHORD

Formation. While embryonic mesoderm formation is taking place, a rod-like structure, the **notochord**, appears in the midline and "appears to grow cranially" from the region of Hensen's node. The exact origin and mechanism of notochord formation in mammals is controversial and appears to be excruciatingly complex. In primitive chordates, however, where its formation is almost diagrammatic in simplicity, the notochord originates as a solid rod-like structure from the roof of the primitive gut (archenteron). For your purposes, start with the notochord in its definitive midline position between the ectoderm and endoderm.

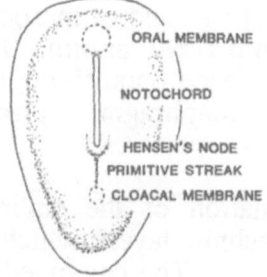

The appearance of the notochord is the first indication of the future axial skeletonand is the most characteristic feature of the phylum to which we belong (Chordata). This structure extends from the caudal edge of the oropharyngeal membrane to the cranial end of the primitive streak (Hensen's node) and plays a major inductive role in the subsequent development of the musculoskeletal and nervous systems.

Fate of the Notochord. After completing its inductive role in the formation of the musculoskeletal and nervous systems, the notochord undergoes regressive changes and disappears in the region of the vertebral bodies but remnants persist in the intervertebral disks as the **nucleus pulposus.** Notochordal remnants may, on rare occasions, give rise to neoplasms called **chordomas.** Almost all of these neoplasms (about 90%) arise in the cranial (basisphenoid) or caudal (sacrococcygeal) regions of the body but they can appear anywhere along the axial skeleton.

QUESTIONS: Chapter 7 - Early Development of the Conceptus

1. The extraembryonic coelomic space is located between the:
   A. syncytiotrophoblast and cytotrophoblast
   B. cytotrophoblast and extraembryonic mesoderm
   C. somatic and splanchnic layers of extraembryonic mesoderm
   D. yolk sac and body stalk
   E. none of the above

2. The primitive streak:
   A. appears near the caudal edge of the bilaminar disk
   B. signifies the onset of embryonic mesoderm formation
   C. appears before the notochord can be identified
   D. determines the body axes of the developing embryo
   E. all of the above

3. The oropharyngeal membrane is located:
   A. between the notochord and primitive streak
   B. immediately caudal to the primitive streak
   C. cranial to the notochord
   D. cranial to the cardiogenic region
   E. between the somatic and splanchnic mesoderm

4. The peripheral limits of the embryonic area (bilaminar and trilaminar) can be identified throughout development by the structures forming the boundaries of the:
   A. oral opening
   B. umbilicus
   C. cloacal membrane
   D. body stalk
   E. embryonic coelom

5. Failure of the embryonic mesoderm to fuse cranial to the oropharyngeal membrane would be expected to interfere with the development of the:
   A. heart
   B. embryonic coelom
   C. septum transversum
   D. anterior body wall above the umbilicus
   E. all of the above

6. Failure of the embryonic mesoderm to fuse caudal to the cloacal membrane would be expected to prevent:
   A. formation of the body stalk
   B. normal development of the abdominal wall below the umbilicus
   C. closure of the primitive streak
   D. formation of the caudal portion of the notochord
   E. all of the above

Answers: 1=C; 2=E; 3=C; 4=B; 5=E; 6=B

CHAPTER 8: DEVELOPMENT OF GENERAL BODY FORM

FOLDING OF THE EMBRYO

Growth in the midline or axial region of the trilaminar embryo is greater than that occurring in peripheral areas and as a consequence, the peripheral areas are gradually overgrown and folded under the central area to form the **body folds**. The division of the conceptus into embryonic and extraembryonic areas, which first became apparent in the bilaminar embryo, is greatly accentuated by the appearance of body folds. The **head fold** is the first to appear and is produced as a result of craniocaudal elongation caused by the rapidly developing notochord and central nervous system; the **tail fold** appears a short time later as a result of the same craniocaudal growth process. Comparable but less distinct **lateral body folds** gradually appear on each side.

With the appearance of the body folds (head, tail and lateral), the flattened trilaminar embryo begins to exhibit the basic tubular configuration of the adult organism. Rapid development of the brain and branchial arches (see below) establishes an easily identifiable head region very early.

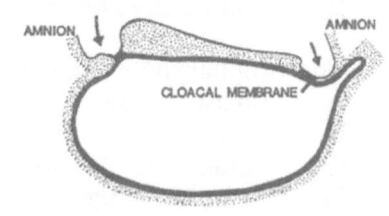

DEVELOPMENT OF GENERAL BODY FORM

It must be emphasized that all components of the trilaminar embryo, i.e., ectoderm, mesoderm (somatic and splanchnic), coelomic spaces and endoderm, participate in the formation of body folds and that the folds themselves establish almost all of the important anatomical relationships seen in the adult.

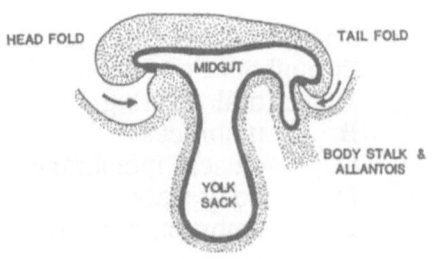

Formation of head and tail folds brings the oropharyngeal and cloacal membranes into their definitive locations on the ventral surface of the body. The development of right and left lateral body folds brings the somatopleure, coelom and splanchnopleure laterally and ventrally to produce the primitive body (somatopleure) and gut (splanchnopleure) walls in the trunk regions between the head and tail folds. The coelomic cavity separating the somatopleure (body wall) and splanchnopleure (gut wall) will eventually form the pericardial, pleural and peritoneal cavities of the adult. Please note that from the time of its appearance in the trilaminar embryo, the embryonic coelom always separates splanchnopleuric structures, e.g., heart (pericardial cavity), lungs (pleural cavity) and digestive tract (peritoneal cavity) from somatopleuric structures, i.e., body wall.

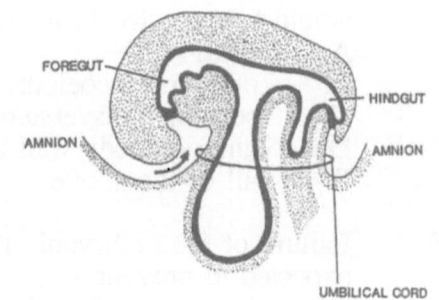

FORMATION OF THE PRIMITIVE GUT

Primitive Foregut: Because the growth processes which produce body folds involve all components of the trilaminar embryo, the head fold contains an endodermal lined tubular prolongation of the yolk sac splanchnopleure; this is the primitive **foregut**. Later in development, the foregut will be divided into dorsal (digestive) and ventral (respiratory) areas. The digestive (dorsal) portion will eventually form the pharynx, esophagus, and stomach; the respiratory (ventral) portion will form the trachea and lungs.

Primitive Midgut: At this time, the midgut is not a complete tubular structure; it possesses a roof and sides but its floor opens via the vitelline duct (yolk stalk) into the main cavity of the yolk sac; later this communication is interrupted and the floor is completed by detachment of the yolk stalk. The midgut splanchnopleure will subsequently form most of the small intestine and part of the colon.

Primitive Hindgut: The tail fold (like the head fold) contains a tubular extension of the yolk sac splanchnopleure which forms the hindgut or cloaca. The hind gut will eventually form the remaining parts of the colon, rectum and urinary bladder. It should be noted that during tail fold formation, the proximal part of the allantois and body stalk move ventrally and cranially and are incorporated into the floor of the hindgut; this is the embryonic or urachal portion of the allantois. Later in development when the cloaca (hindgut) is divided into dorsal (rectal) and ventral (urogenital) areas, the urachal portion of the allantois is attached to the cranial end of the urogenital sinus, i.e., urinary bladder.

BRANCHIAL ARCHES

The pharyngeal region of the foregut is characterized by the formation of branchial or pharyngeal arches. These paired structures are incompletely-separated, vertical columns of body wall. The arches are covered externally by ectoderm, internally by endoderm and each possesses a core of embryonic mesenchyme which is usually categorized as branchiomeric mesenchyme. Externally, adjacent arches are separated by branchial grooves which correspond in position to internally located pharyngeal pouches. The subsequent fate of each pair of branchial arches is complex but an understanding of their differentiation is essential for understanding head and neck development. The first pair of arches develop around the oropharyngeal membrane. Later developmental changes convert these arches into the upper and lower jaws. Branchial arch differentiation will be covered in special sections devoted to the branchial apparatus.

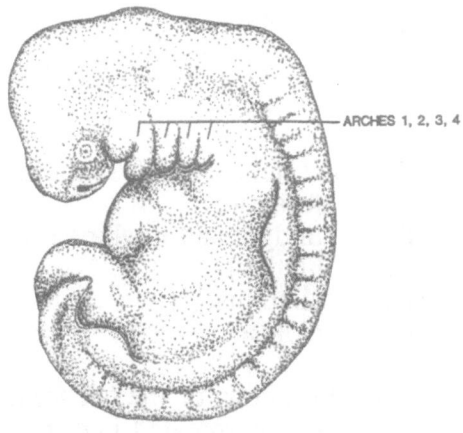

BRANCHIAL ARCHES

ARCHES 1, 2, 3, 4

QUESTIONS: Chapter 8 - Development of General Body Form

1. Conversion of the trilaminar embryonic plate into a tubular configuration is accomplished by the appearance of the:
   A. primitive streak
   B. notochord
   C. body folds
   D. body stalk
   E. prochordal plate

2. All of the following are moved ventrally and caudally during head fold formation **EXCEPT** the:
   A. septum transversum
   B. notochord
   C. oral membrane
   D. pericardial cavity
   E. heart

3. Which of the following is **NOT** moved ventrally and cranially during formation of the tail fold?
   A. primitive streak
   B. allantois
   C. cloacal membrane
   D. placental blood vessels
   E. notochord

4. Which structure is **NOT** produced as a direct result of body fold formation?
   A. foregut
   B. midgut and vitelline (yolk) duct
   C. hindgut
   D. allantois
   E. cloaca

5. After formation of the tail fold, the proximal part of the allantois:
   A. is incorporated into the hindgut
   B. has luminal continuity with the cloaca
   C. is located ventral to the embryo
   D. is located at the cranial end of the cloaca
   E. all of the above

6. The tubular configuration of the early embryo is produced as a result of folds appearing in the:
   A. somatopleura
   B. splanchnopleura
   C. both
   D. neither

Answers: 1=C; 2=B; 3=E; 4=D; 5=E; 6=C

CHAPTER 9: NERVOUS SYSTEM

NEURAL TUBE FORMATION

The presence of a notochord is necessary for initiating development of the nervous system, however, complete histological differentiation also requires the presence of segmented paraxial mesoderm (somites).

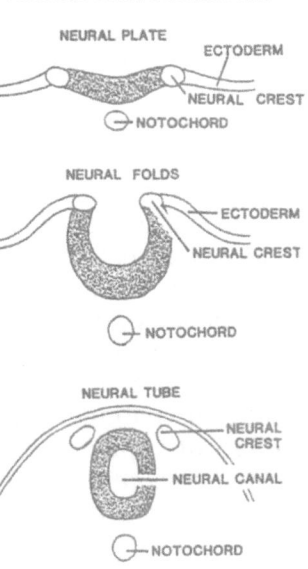

The nervous system makes its first appearance as a thickening in the ectodermal cells (neural plate) over the notochord. The **neural plate** is converted into a tubular structure by a folding-fusing process which separates the presumptive **neural ectoderm** from the adjacent **integumentary ectoderm**. Complete fusion of the neural folds is necessary for normal development because this allows the mesodermal components which form meninges, bone, muscle and skin to reach the dorsal midline over the neural tube.

EARLY DEVELOPMENTAL DEFECTS

Failure of the neural folds to fuse dorsally (myeloschisis) is one of the most common and severe developmental defects of the central nervous system. Failure of the neural folds to fuse produces an extreme range of developmental defects which of necessity also includes major defects in the associated mesodermal components (meninges, neural arches, epimeric musculature, skin) which normally cover the dorsal aspect of the neural tube. The spectrum of defects between **complete craniosacral myeloschisis to spina bifida occulta** includes the meningocele and meningomyelocele complexes (spina bifida cystica). The entire series of defects can be explained by failure or delayed fusion of the folds since delayed fusion disrupts normal development of all associated structures (meninges, bone, muscle, skin). It should be noted that if the neural folds fail to fuse at any level, the neural tissue at that level ceases to develop and undergoes regressive changes to produce a thin transparent membrane devoid of neural elements. **Anencephaly** is caused by failure of the neural folds to fuse in the cranial region and is incompatible with extrauterine survival; it is also frequently associated with **polyhydramnios** because the absence of a swallowing reflex interferes with amniotic fluid exchange. Comparable lesions at lower levels are usually compatible with extrauterine survival but are associated with paralysis below the lesion; the type of paralysis depends on the extent and location of the lesion. Neural tube defects involving the brain (anencephaly) and cystic varieties of spina bifida can usually be diagnosed in utero with ultrasound scan because these defects produce characteristic changes in the outline of the fetal image. Open neural tubes defects can be detected by analyzing amniotic fluid for alpha-fetoprotein; levels in amniotic fluid are very high both in the cystic and noncystic forms.

NEURAL TUBE DEFECTS MAY AFFECT NEURAL CREST CELL FORMATION

Pre-fusion defects of the neural tube which interfere with the formation of neural crest cells (ectomesenchyme) may also be associated with a wide variety of non-neural defects in the head and neck. Neural crest mesenchyme (ectomesenchyme) is known to form the major portion of all connective tissue elements found in the head and neck. Cranial and facial defects which are currently attributed to deficiencies in mesenchyme formation by neural crest cells include: agenesis and/or hypoplasia of bones forming the face. The latter group includes the severe facial abnormalities of premaxillary agenesis, agnathia (mandibular agenesis), otocephaly and cebocephaly.

PERIPHERAL NERVOUS SYSTEM: SPINAL AND CRANIAL NERVES

The development and distribution of nervous elements (ganglia and nerves) in the somatic division of the peripheral nervous system is intimately associated with skeletal muscle that develops from somites or in association with branchial arches. Individual myogenic cells (muscle forming) frequently migrate to positions far beyond their site of origin before differentiating into histologically recognizable skeletal muscle fibers. The origin and course of their motor (efferent) nerves indicate their original position and the migratory pathway followed in reaching their final destination.

SPINAL AND CRANIAL NERVES

The primary sensory neurons for all spinal and most cranial nerves appear to be derived from an intermediate zone of ectoderm between the developing neural folds and adjacent integumentary ectoderm. During neural fold fusion, this intermediate zone of ectoderm is carried below the surface ectoderm but is not incorporated into the neural tube proper. These cells remain as a dorsal strip of neuroectodermal cells along each side of the newly formed tube and are referred to as the **neural crest cells**. A short time later, the neural crest becomes discontinuous to form the primordia for the **sensory ganglia** of spinal and branchiomeric cranial nerves. Differentiating primary sensory neurons are originally **bipolar** with central and peripheral processes; the centrally directed process enters the developing neural tube dorsally and eventually forms synaptic connections with secondary sensory neurons which receive, integrate and relay incoming (afferent) information to other parts of the spinal cord and brain. In **mixed cranial nerves** (branchiomeric), the peripheral processes immediately join the dorsally emerging motor fibers to form the mixed trunk of the main nerve. In **mixed spinal nerves**, the peripheral processes join the ventrally emerging motor fibers after a short independent course to form the mixed part of the main nerve. (For significance of dorsal and ventral exit of motor fibers see Branchiomeric Musculature in the following chapter). During later stages of histological differentiation, the central and peripheral processes of the bipolar sensory neurons are brought into apposition to produce the definitive **unipolar** neurons found in almost all sensory ganglia. Some of the neural crest cells within the developing ganglia differentiate into the **Schwann** and **satellite cells** ensheathing all parts of the peripheral nervous system (myelinated and nonmyelinated). Other neural crest cells migrate to distant sites to form neuroblasts and Schwann cells for the autonomic (sympathetic and parasympathetic) ganglia. Migratory neural crest cells are also known to form or contribute to the formation of the following non-neural elements:

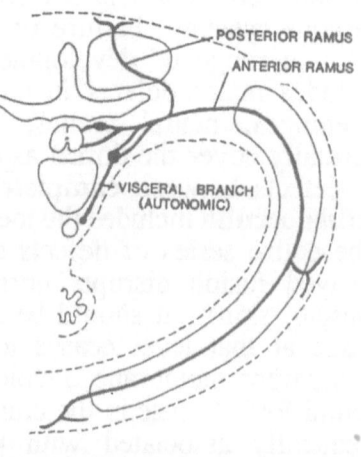

PERIPHERAL NERVE DEVELOPMENT

POSTERIOR RAMUS

ANTERIOR RAMUS

VISCERAL BRANCH (AUTONOMIC)

1. pigment cells of the skin (melanocytes).
2. teeth (except the enamel).
3. many bones of the skull and face (ectomesenchyme).
4. chromaffin cells of the adrenal medulla.

PERIPHERAL NERVOUS SYSTEM: AUTONOMICS

SYMPATHETIC (THORACOLUMBAR) DIVISION

Cells originating from the neural crest migrate ventrally to reach positions adjacent to the developing vertebral bodies and subsequently differentiate into neurons of the paravertebral sympathetic **chain ganglia**. Other neural crest cells continue their ventral migration to the anterior surface of the vertebrae, surround the dorsal aorta and differentiate into neurons of the periaortic **collateral ganglia**. These two groups of ganglia constitute the major concentrations of sympathetic postganglionic neurons. Chromaffin cells, e.g., adrenal medulla, which are modified postganglionic neurons are sometimes listed separately as a third group. Chain ganglia are relatively constant in size, number and location but the collateral ganglia are extremely variable. Because of their variability, the collateral ganglia are named by their proximity to major arterial branches of the dorsal aorta, e.g., celiac, aorticorenal, mesenteric (superior and inferior), intermesenteric and hypogastric ganglia.

Chain Ganglia. During the early stages of development, the number of chain ganglia formed on each side corresponds to the number of developing spinal ganglia, i.e., thirty-one. A short time later, two sympathetic nerves develop in association with each chain ganglion; these sympathetic nerves are the thirty-one **gray rami communicantes** and **visceral sympathetic nerves**.

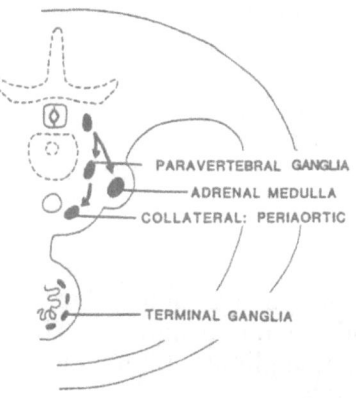

AUTONOMIC NERVOUS SYSTEM

PARAVERTEBRAL GANGLIA
ADRENAL MEDULLA
COLLATERAL: PERIAORTIC

TERMINAL GANGLIA

Gray Rami Communicantes. Neural continuity between somatic peripheral nerves (spinal) and sympathetic chain ganglia is provided by the gray rami. Despite subsequent fusion of some chain ganglia, all thirty-one gray rami retain their identity and can be identified easily in the adult. **Gray rami provide sympathetic innervation for structures located in the body wall (somatopleura) and are always postganglionic.**

Visceral Sympathetic Nerves. Neural continuity between the two groups of sympathetic ganglia (chain and collateral) is provided by the segmentally arranged visceral sympathetic nerves. Individual nerves may be **preganglionic, postganglionic or both**; preganglionic fibers will ultimately synapse in one of the collateral ganglia. Visceral nerves do not innervate visceral structures directly; instead, all enter and participate in forming the great, nerve plexus (sympathetic and parasympathetic) surrounding the dorsal aorta. Sympathetic innervation for splanchnopleuric structures located in the thorax, abdomen and pelvis is derived from corresponding levels of the aortic plexus, e.g., heart and lungs via the cardiac and pulmonary plexi of the thoracic aorta; gut via the plexus of the abdominal aorta; pelvic viscera via the hypogastric plexus. It should be noted that the middle sacral artery is the direct continuation of the embryonic dorsal aorta; the hypogastric plexus represents the pelvic or sacral level of the aortic plexus.

Note: It is not widely appreciated that visceral sympathetic nerves are segmentally arranged and that all thirty-one persist in the adult; their abundance and regularity is usually unrecognized because the names assigned to the definitive nerves do not reflect their common origin. The accompanying list gives the segmental origin and names for the adult sympathetic visceral nerves.

C	1-4	superior cervical sympathetic cardiac nerve
C	5-6	middle cervical sympathetic cardiac nerve
C	7-8	inferior cervical sympathetic nerve
T	1-4	thoracic cardiac nerves (four separate nerves)
		(also called upper thoracic splanchnic nerves)
T	5-9	greater splanchnic nerve
T	10-11	lesser splanchnic nerve
T	12	least splanchnic nerve (variable)
L	1-5	lumbar splanchnic nerves (4-5 separate nerves)
S	1-5	sacral splanchnic nerves (2-4 separate nerves)

Visceral nerves provide sympathetic innervation for structures originating from the splanchnopleure; preganglionic fibers may synapse either in chain ganglia or in periaortic collateral ganglia.

Sympathetic Trunk.   Neural continuity between the central nervous system and the sympathetic nervous system occurs only at thoracic and upper lumbar levels of the spinal cord. Continuity is established when efferent fibers from fourteen segments of the spinal cord (TI-L2) reach the chain ganglia; these communicating nerve fibers are the preganglionic **white rami communicantes.** After reaching the chain ganglia (thoracic and upper lumbar), some of the fibers grow cranially through adjacent ganglia to supply preganglionic fibers for the cervical chain ganglia; other fibers grow caudally to supply preganglionic fibers for the lower lumbar and sacral ganglia. The **sympathetic trunk** is formed by the appearance of these interganglionic fibers (ascending and descending) between the segmentally arranged chain ganglia.

PARASYMPATHETIC (CRANIOSACRAL) DIVISION

Neuroblasts forming the **terminal ganglia** for the parasympathetic division of the peripheral nervous system originate from neural crest cells located at cranial or sacral levels (S2-4) of the neural tube.

Cranial Terminal Ganglia.   In the head, four terminal parasympathetic ganglia occur regularly, i.e., **ciliary, submandibular, pterygopalatine** and **otic.** All of the cranial ganglia are constant in position, anatomically well defined, located near the organs innervated and all receive their preganglionic fibers either from the oculomotor (ciliary), the facial (submandibular and pterygopalatine) or the glossopharyngeal (otic) nerves.

Trunk Terminal Ganglia.   In trunk regions of the body, terminal ganglia are inconstant in position, diffuse and located on or within (intrinsic ganglia) the walls of the organs innervated. Distribution of parasympathetic fibers in the trunk is limited entirely or almost entirely to visceral structures originating from the splanchnopleure; spinal nerves which innervate somatopleuric structures do not contain parasympathetic fibers.

Above the descending colon, the diffuse intrinsic ganglia of the digestive tract (Meissner's and Auerbach's) receive their preganglionic fibers from **splanchnic (visceral) branches of the vagus** distributed via the nerve plexus of the aorta. Near the splenic flexure, the intrinsic ganglia begin to receive preganglionic fibers from the **pelvic splanchnic nerves** directly, i.e., visceral branches are not distributed via the aortic plexus. The unnamed terminal ganglia of the urogenital system also receive their preganglionic fibers from the pelvic splanchnic nerves. Do not confuse pelvic splanchnic nerves (parasympathetic) with sacral splanchnic nerves (sympathetic).

CENTRAL NERVOUS SYSTEM

Immediately after its formation, the neuroectodermal cells forming the wall of the neural tube are arranged in the form of a pseudostratified columnar epithelium surrounding a central **neural canal**. Internally, the apex of these cells exhibit well developed junctional complexes which are visualized microscopically as the **internal limiting membrane**; externally, the basal cytoplasm is attached to the basal lamina (basement membrane) which forms the **external limiting membrane** (future pia-glial membrane). Cellular proliferation within the lateral walls of the neural tube soon results in stratification and the appearance of two incompletely separated cell populations which are referred to as the **ependymal** (periventricular) and **mantle** zones or layers.

DEVELOPMENT OF GRAY AND WHITE MATTER

Ependymal Layer. Cells forming the innermost periventricular zone possess junctional complexes and surround the neural canal; descendants of these cells (with junctional complexes) will surround the neural canal and all of its derivatives (brain ventricles) throughout life. Most of the ependymal progeny however, do not possess junctional complexes and accumulate laterally to form the population of cells known as the **mantle layer.** Ependymal or periventricular cells are **mitotically active** (germinal) throughout intrauterine development and are the ultimate source of all neurons and macroglia found in the central nervous system.

Mantle Layer. The laterally dispersed cells forming the mantle zone are primitive **neuroblasts** and **glioblasts.** Although glial cells retain the capacity to divide throughout life, neuroblasts do not divide after entering the mantle layer and as a consequence the ependymal (periventricular) cells must continue to produce new neuroblasts until the full complement of adult neurons has been attained, i.e., until or shortly after birth. As neurons differentiate within the mantle layer, their processes (axons) begin to accumulate near the external limiting membrane to produce an area which is almost totally devoid of cell nuclei; this area is the **marginal layer.** The mantle layer is the presumptive **gray matter** for all parts of the spinal cord and brain.

Marginal Layer. The marginal layer thickens rapidly as additional axons are added from neurons developing in the underlying mantle layer and from the centrally directed processes of primary sensory neurons located in the ganglia of cranial and spinal nerves. Later, the thickness and prominence of the marginal layer will be greatly enhanced by the differentiation of oligodendroglial cells and the appearance of myelin. The marginal layer is the presumptive **white matter** for all parts of the spinal cord and brain.

With the appearance of the marginal layer, the basic morphological pattern for the distribution of gray (neuron cell bodies) and white (nerve cell processes) matter in the CNS is established. During subsequent stages of CNS differentiation, this basic distribution pattern of central gray and peripheral white matter is modified in only two areas of the brain. In these areas, an external layer of gray matter appears superficial to the white or marginal layer; this external layer of gray matter forms the **cortex** of the cerebrum and cerebellum. Cortical neurons and glia, like those of the central gray, are derived from the underlying ependymal layer.

Vascularization of the Neural Tube. Initially, fibers of the marginal layer accumulate between the basal cytoplasm of the ependymal or periventricular cells which extends from the internal to the external limiting membrane. At this time, the nuclei of these elongated germinal cells migrate regularly between the limiting membranes; migration is necessary because the neural tube, an epithelial derivative, is avascular and the nearest blood vessels are adjacent to the external limiting membrane. Nuclei migrate peripherally during the synthetic and growth phases of their life cycle but move centrally to undergo mitosis thereby providing vascular access to the migrating nuclei of other germinal cells. After dividing, one daughter cell retains contact with both surface membranes and its nucleus continues to migrate; the other daughter cell enters the mantle layer as a primitive neuroblast and ceases to divide. Some time later, blood vessels from the developing **pia mater** penetrate and vascularize all parts of the neural tube so that migration is no longer necessary. After vascularization, most of the germinal cells lose their connections with the external membrane. In thin areas of the adult CNS, ependymal cells which have, retained both connections can still be identified. The appearance of **microglia** is reported to coincide with vascularization.

DEVELOPMENT OF SENSORY AND MOTOR REGIONS

Functional Differentiation. Manifestations of functional differentiation appear in the neural tube before histological differentiation of the presumptive gray (mantle) and white (marginal) matter is complete. The onset of functional differentiation is indicated by the appearance of an internal longitudinal groove in the lateral walls of the neural tube; this important landmark is the **sulcus limitans** and it is used to divide the lateral walls of the neural tube into dorsal and ventral areas which are referred to, respectively, as the **alar** and **basal plates**.

Alar plates (dorsal) are concerned with sensory function and all secondary sensory neurons (which receive, integrate and relay afferent information) are located in the dorsal gray matter of the spinal cord and brain.

Basal plates (ventral) are concerned with motor functions and all efferent neurons (which respond with the appropriate motor response) are located in the ventral gray matter of the spinal cord and brain.

It is important to note that the alar and basal plates possess all three layers of the neural tube (ependyma, mantle, marginal) but that the right and left sides are connected across the midline by ependyma only. The ependymal membrane connecting the dorsal edges of the alar plates forms the roof or **dorsal lamina** of the neural tube; that between the ventral edges of the basal plates forms the floor or **ventral lamina**. The ependymal membranes forming the dorsal and ventral lamina are very important because all fibers crossing the midline (decussations and commissures) must utilize either the dorsal or ventral lamina.

All levels of the neural tube caudal to the forebrain contain alar (sensory) and basal (motor) plates which are demarcated by the sulcus limitans; forebrain areas (telencephalon and diencephalon) possess only the alar or sensory component.

DIFFERENTIATION OF THE SPINAL CORD

The structural organization of the three layered neural tube and the adult spinal cord are shown in the accompanying illustration. Each structure possesses a centrally located neural canal surrounded by ependyma, an intermediate layer of mantle cells (gray matter), and a superficial marginal layer of nerve cell processes (white matter).

In the adult cord, the gray matter (mantle) is arranged in the shape of the letter "H" to produce the **anterior** and **posterior gray columns**. The dorsal and ventral extensions are produced during subsequent stages of development by the addition of mantle neuroblasts and by the differentiation of nerve cell bodies (perikarya). The perikarya of motor neurons in the anterior gray column are much larger than those of the dorsally located secondary sensory neurons: this difference is reflected by the greater size of the anterior gray column. The "H-shaped" gray matter is used to demarcate areas of the marginal layer (now myelinated) as the dorsal, lateral and ventral **white columns**. Ventrally, the median floor area has remained thin and is associated with the **anterior sulcus**. A slight thickening in this area has been produced by encroachment of the adjacent gray (mantle) and ventral crossing (decussation) of a few fibers in the ventral ependymal lamina. Dorsally, the ependymal lamina is greatly thickened and is associated with a shallow median groove rather than a deep sulcus. Initially, a dorsal sulcus is present but as the posterior white columns increase in size, the lateral walls are brought into apposition and the sulcus is gradually obliterated. The position of the dorsal sulcus in the adult is indicated by a midline depression and a few remnants of pia forming the indistinct **dorsal median septum**. Dorsal thickening in the spinal cord is the result of encroachment rather than fiber decussation in the dorsal ependymal lamina.

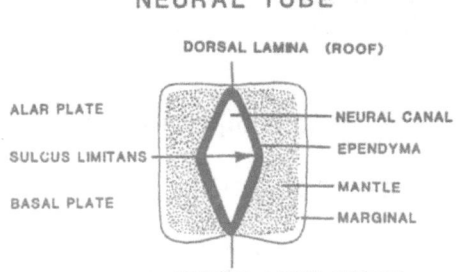

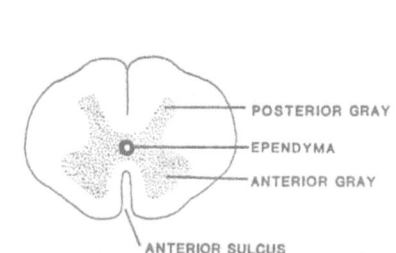

DIFFERENTIATION OF THE BRAIN

Early development of the encephalon is indicated by the appearance of three primitive brain vesicles. In craniocaudal sequence, the primitive brain vesicles are the: **prosencephalon, mesencephalon** and **rhombencephalon**.

Subdivision of the prosencephalon produces the definitive telencephalic and diencephalic portions of the adult forebrain; the primitive mesencephalon remains undivided and persists to become the definitive mesencephalon or midbrain; the rhombencephalon is divided by the pontine flexure into the metencephalic and myelencephalic portions of the adult hindbrain. The most important gross structures developing from or associated with the definitive brain vesicles are listed below.

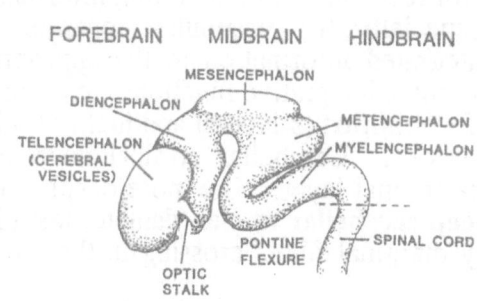

1. Telencephalon - cerebral vesicles
2. Diencephalon - thalamus, hypothalamus, neurohypophysis, pineal and retina
3. Mesencephalon - superior and inferior colliculi and cerebral peduncles
4. Metencephalon - cerebellum and pons
5. Myelencephalon - medulla

Note: One of the most striking changes seen at brain levels of the neural tube is the apparent loss of anterior and posterior gray columns which characterize the alar and basal plate areas of the spinal cord. Although the classical "H-shaped" configuration of the central gray is not seen in the brain, the corresponding sensory and motor neurons persist as "discontinuous gray columns" which form the various sensory and motor nuclei of cranial nerves. Cranial nerve nuclei which subserve different modalities (sensory or motor) retain their alar or basal plate locations in the adult.

To simplify the changes converting the neural tube into the adult brain, the sequence of presentation will begin with the myelencephalon and progress cranially to the telencephalon.

Myelencephalon.   The medulla retains much of the basic structural arrangement seen at spinal levels. The major change is separation or flaring of the alar plates and stretching of the thin ependymal membrane forming the dorsal lamina. The flaring, which is responsible for displacing the sulcus limitans to the floor of the neural canal, is attributed to the pontine flexure. The expanded ependymal lamina of the roof and the adjacent layer of pia (tela choroidea) form the **choroid plexus** of the fourth ventricle; subsequent degenerations laterally and in the midline form, respectively, the foramina of **Luschka** and **Magendie**.

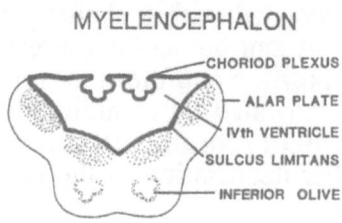

Basal Plate.   Motor nuclei of cranial nerves XII, X-XI (vagal complex) and IX.

Alar Plate.   Sensory nuclei (secondary sensory neurons) for cranial nerves X and IX.

The ventral ependymal lamina is greatly thickened and the anterior sulcus is eliminated by ventral decussation of marginal fiber tracts, i.e., **pyramidal decussation.** The enlarged neural canal forms the caudal part of the fourth ventricle.

Metencephalon.   The metencephalon is associated with the development of two very large structures (cerebellum and pons) which superficially at least, obscure the basic tubular pattern of the CNS. The cerebellum is formed by enormous development and fusion of the alar plates. The massive growth is associated with receiving and integrating information from multiple sources (especially the vestibular apparatus) and then relaying the integrated information to the appropriate motor areas. These complex integrative functions are accompanied by the appearance

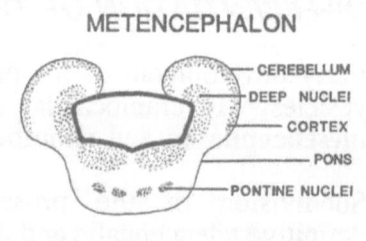

of a stratified (3 layers) and highly folded cortex (superficial gray) to accommodate the required neurons. Cerebellar cortical neurons (**Purkinje and granule cells**) are derived from the ependymal layer. The more deeply placed alar mantle cells contribute to the formation of the **deep cerebellar nuclei** (dentate, fastigial, emboliform, globose). The pons is formed primarily by marginal fibers crossing in the ependymal lamina of the floor.

Basal Plate.   Motor nuclei of cranial nerves VII, VI and V.

Alar Plate.   Sensory nuclei (secondary sensory neurons) for cranial nerves VIII, VII and V; the vestibular nuclei of VIII are unusually large.

The neural canal contributes to the formation of the cranial part of the fourth ventricle.

Mesencephalon.   The midbrain retains most of the basic structure of the neural tube seen at the spinal levels.

Basal Plate.   Motor nuclei of cranial nerves IV and III.

Alar Plate.   Neurons located in the collicular area perform integrative functions for coordinating eye movements only, i.e., they are not secondary sensory neurons for cranial nerves IV and III; these nerves do not possess ganglia.

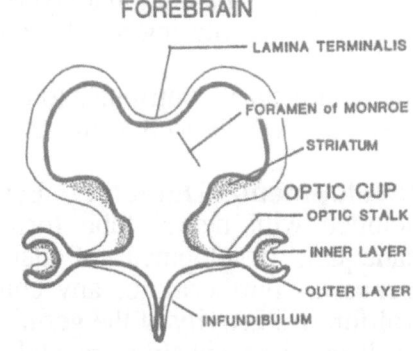

MESENCEPHALON
- SUPERIOR COLLICULUS
- AQUEDUCT OF SYLVIUS
- RED NUCLEUS
- SUBSTIANTA NIGRA
- CEREBRAL PEDUNCLE

Note: In lower vertebrates, the visual cortex is located in the collicular area of the midbrain and these animals "see" with their mesencephalon.   In higher vertebrates, optic fibers are relayed anteriorly to the visual cortex of the cerebrum, i.e., occipital lobes; higher vertebrates "see" with their telencephalon. Neurons of the old mesencephalic visual cortex now perform integrative functions for coordinating eye movements.   Remnants of the primitive stratified visual cortex can be identified in the human collicular area.

The cerebral peduncles are localized thickenings in the marginal layer produced by the large numbers of fibers entering and leaving the forebrain areas.   The neural canal persists as the **aqueduct of Sylvius.**

Diencephalon.   Currently, the diencephalon is considered to contain only the alar components of the neural tube.   At one time, however, the hypothalamic sulcus, which appears to be a cranial extension of the sulcus limitans, was used to divide the diencephalon into classical alar and basal plates.

Gross structures derived from the diencephalic alar plates and the ependymal lamina include the thalamus, hypothalamus, epiphysis (pineal), neurohypophysis and retina.   During subsequent developmental stages, most of the diencephalic vesicle becomes buried by caudal growth of the telencephalon.

Thalamic and **hypothalamic nuclei** originate from the mantle of the buried portion of the diencephalon; the **pineal** and **neurohypophysis** originate from the thin ependymal laminae joining the upper and lower portions of the alar plates.

Retina.   The visual part of the retina develops directly from the wall of the diencephalon and although it is highly specialized, the inner layer of the optic cup exhibits the basic, three layered organization of the neural tube.   The photoreceptor cells (rods and cones) are modified ependymal cells with junctional complexes; the retinal neurons (bipolar, horizontal, amacrine, ganglionic) and glia (Muller's cells) are derived from the mantle layer; the nerve fiber layer is comparable to the marginal layer of white matter found elsewhere.   Neuroectodermal cells forming the outer layer of the optic cup do not proliferate to produce a mantle layer but persist and form the pigmented layer of the definitive retina.   It should be noted that the optic nerve (II) is a fiber tract (marginal derivative) rather than a true peripheral nerve with Schwann cells; decussating fibers of the optic nerve (chiasma) cross the midline in the thin ependymal membrane joining the lower edges of the diencephalic alar plates.

FOREBRAIN
- LAMINA TERMINALIS
- FORAMEN of MONROE
- STRIATUM
- OPTIC CUP
- OPTIC STALK
- INNER LAYER
- OUTER LAYER
- INFUNDIBULUM

Telencephalon. The telencephalon is the highest integrative center of the brain and like the diencephalon, it contains only the alar component of the neural tube. The most cranial limits of the ependymal membrane joining the right and left alar plates is referred to as the **lamina terminalis** and is associated with the formation of cerebral commissures, i.e., anterior hippocampal and corpus callosum. The complex integrative functions of the telencephalon can be correlated with the presence of a multilayered neocortex (6 layers), exceedingly large, bilateral hemispheres and the appearance of sulci and gyri; its only nerve is the olfactory (I) which originates as multiple rootlets from the bipolar neurons located in the olfactory mucosa. The cortical neurons (pyramidal cells) and glia originate from the underlying germinal ependyma; the deeper mantle neurons of the **corpus striatum** contribute to the formation of the basal ganglia (caudate and lentiform nuclei).

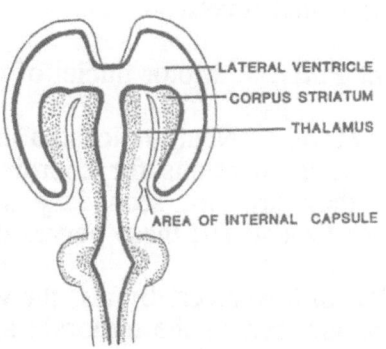

TELENCEPHALON

LATERAL VENTRICLE
CORPUS STRIATUM
THALAMUS
AREA OF INTERNAL CAPSULE

Three unusually prominent fiber bundles (marginal derivatives) are associated with the cerebral vesicles.

1. The **corpus callosum** crosses the midline to connect the right and left cerebral hemispheres and is so large that the thin ependymal membrane of the lamina terminalis is stretched inferiorly to cover the dorsal aspect of the diencephalon and part of the mesencephalon.

2. The **hippocampal commissure** (body of the fornix) crosses the midline below corpus callosum and although it is of considerable size, it appears small in comparison to the corpus callosum.

3. The **internal capsule** is a very large fiber tract rather than a commissure and represents the apposed marginal layers of the diencephalon and telencephalon. The two marginal layers are brought into apposition by caudal expansion of the cerebral vesicle and overgrowth of the diencephalon. The combined marginal layers form the internal capsule which separates the mantle derivatives of the telencephalon (caudate and lentiform nuclei) from the mantle derivatives of the diencephalon (thalamus). The marginal layers do not fuse; the cleft separating the marginal layers is gradually obliterated by the massive accumulation of fibers entering and leaving the developing cerebral hemispheres and thalamic areas.

The neural canal contributes to the formation of the cranial part of the third ventricle; the lateral extensions which accompany the vesicles form the **lateral ventricles**.

Developmental Defects. Early fusion defects, e.g., myeloschisis, anencephaly, etc., were included with neural tube formation. A wide variety of CNS defects may result from inadequate development of alar and basal plate derivatives at any level, e.g., cerebellar agenesis. Furthermore, any condition (genetic or environmental) which interferes with the proliferative activity of the germinal ependyma at any time during intrauterine development may result in microcephaly or mental retardation. Developmental defects of the forebrain involving absence of bilaterality, e.g., holoprosencephaly, arrhinencephaly, agenesis of the corpus callosum, etc., are thought to originate with abnormal development or displacement of the olfactory placodes. The midline (median) forebrain anomalies are usually associated with severe facial abnormalities which may involve the interorbital areas, e.g. cyclopia, median clefts of the lip.

QUESTIONS: Chapter 9 - Nervous System

1. Which statement best describes development of the neural tube?
   A. It develops by dorsal fusion of the neural crest cells.
   B. It develops directly from the primitive streak.
   C. It develops directly from the notochord.
   D. It develops from ectoderm immediately dorsal to the notochord.
   E. It develops from ectoderm immediately dorsal to the primitive streak.

2. Failure of the neural folds to fuse in the dorsal midline at spinal levels invariably produces associated defects in all of the following **EXCEPT** the:
   A. meninges
   B. vertebral body
   C. skin
   D. axial musculature
   E. neural arch processes (vertebral arches)

3. The alar and basal plate areas of the developing central nervous system are separated by the:
   A. sulcus limitans
   B. anterior spinal sulcus
   C. marginal layer
   D. mantle layer
   E. primitive streak

4. Neurons in the central nervous system develop:
   A. in the alar plate
   B. in the basal plate
   C. in the mantle layer
   D. from cells in the periventricular zone (ependymal layer)
   E. all of the above

5. Which of the following is **NOT** derived from neural crest cells?
   A. dorsal root ganglion cells
   B. adrenal medullary cells
   C. Schwann cells
   D. oligodendroglial cells
   E. trigeminal ganglion cells

6. Motor neurons innervating skeletal muscles differentiate from neuroblasts located in the:
   A. alar plate mantle layer
   B. basal plate mantle layer
   C. lateral cell column
   D. alar plate marginal layer
   E. basal plate marginal layer

Answers: 1=D; 2=B; 3=A; 4=E; 5=D; 6=B

CHAPTER 10: MUSCULOSKELETAL SYSTEM

EMBRYONIC MESODERM

PARAXIAL MESODERM

The part of the embryonic mesoderm immediately adjacent to the notochord is referred to as the **paraxial mesoderm**: it extends caudally from the oropharyngeal membrane to the level of the primitive streak (future coccygeal region). During subsequent stages of development, almost all of the paraxial mesoderm will undergo a series of craniocaudal condensations to form the segmentally arranged **somites**.

Somite Formation.   The first pair of somites appears in the paraxial mesoderm about the twenty-first day of development; somite pairs continue to appear at the rate of three per day until approximately 40 ± 4 pairs are formed (4 occipital, 8 cervical, 12 thoracic, 5 lumbar, 5 sacral and 8-10 coccygeal). Historically, the most cephalic somites are considered atypical and are usually referred to as the preotic somites (3 pairs) rather than being numbered.   Recent studies have suggested that all paraxial mesoderm cranial to the occipital somites becomes incompletely segmented to form 7 somitomeres. The 7 somitomeres and 4 occipital somites contribute to the formation of the head and branchial apparatus. Only 31 pairs of the post-cranial somites will

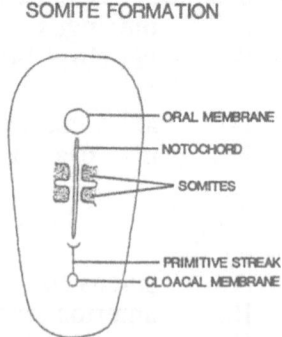

SOMITE FORMATION

- ORAL MEMBRANE
- NOTOCHORD
- SOMITES
- PRIMITIVE STREAK
- CLOACAL MEMBRANE

persist and make significant contributions to the definitive axial skeleton and body musculature; the excess caudal somites regress. The number of persisting somites will also be reflected by the number of spinal nerves induced to develop; the caudal somites regress before spinal nerve development is initiated. Typical somites found in the post-cranial region consist of three parts: **sclerotome**, **myotome** and **dermatome**.

Sclerotomes are the skeletal forming portions of somites and each sclerotome will contribute to the formation of the vertebrae, intervertebral disks, ribs and sternum of the axial skeleton.

Myotomes are the muscle forming portions of somites and they will form **all** of the skeletal muscle found in the post-cranial body wall and appendages; all of these muscles will be innervated by motor fibers in the ventral roots of spinal nerves.

Dermatomes are the integumentary (dermis forming) portions of somites but they do not appear to be independent, self-differentiation units in humans and other mammals; their role in the differentiation of integumentary structures cannot be separated from the myotome.

The **cephalic paraxial mesoderm**, which is partially segmented into seven pairs of **somitomeres**, has the **same developmental potential as a somite**, although no distinct myotome, sclerotome or dermatome regions develop.

INTERMEDIATE MESODERM

The **intermediate mesoderm** is a narrow zone of nonsegmented mesoderm joining the medially located somites with the laterally located lateral plate mesoderm. Intermediate mesoderm is subsequently involved in the formation of the urinary and reproductive system and is sometimes referred to as the **nephrotome**.

LATERAL PLATE MESODERM

The embryonic mesoderm located lateral to the intermediate mesoderm is referred to as the **lateral plate mesoderm.** Initially, the lateral plate is coextensive with the paraxial mesoderm, but the plate rapidly extends cranially and caudally, fuses across the midline and eventually surrounds all of the axial structures of the embryo (oropharyngeal membrane, notochord, primitive streak and cloacal membrane). Embryonic coelom formation soon separates the lateral plate into **somatic** and **splanchnic layers** which form the boundaries for all parts of the coelomic space (pericardial, pleural, peritoneal). The somatic and splanchnic layers become associated with the adjacent ectodermal and endodermal epithelium to form the **somatopleura** and **splanchnopleura**, i.e., the primitive body and gut walls, respectively.

Note: The absence of a coelomic space in the mesenchyme of the head and neck region is explained by formation of the head fold. Most of the mesenchyme appearing in the region of the pharyngeal foregut (future head and neck) develops after head fold formation is well advanced and the most cephalic portion of the embryo and coelom (pericardial cavity) has been folded ventrally and caudally. As a consequence of its late formation and absence of a coelomic space, the mesenchyme in this area remains as a single unsplit layer which (because of its location) is referred to as the **branchiomeric mesenchyme.** A short time later, five ectodermally lined branchial grooves will appear in this area and delineate the external boundaries of the branchial arches.

Note: The appearance of somites within the paraxial mesoderm is used as the basis for classifying embryonic mesoderm as either **segmented** or **unsegmented.**

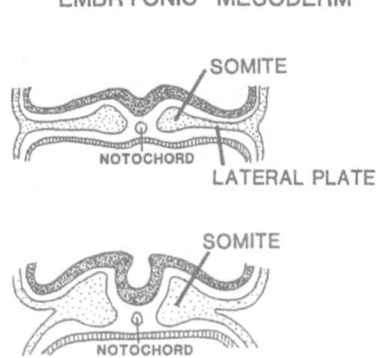

EMBRYONIC MESODERM

SOMITE

NOTOCHORD

LATERAL PLATE

SOMITE

NOTOCHORD

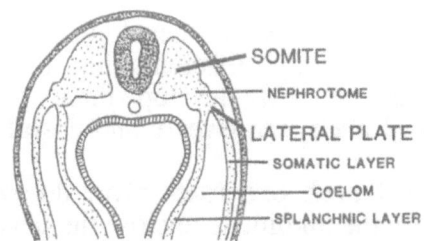

SOMITE

NEPHROTOME

LATERAL PLATE

SOMATIC LAYER

COELOM

SPLANCHNIC LAYER

> **Segmented (somitic) mesoderm** is a very specific term used to indicate tissues and structures developing from somites. (Please note spelling: som**i**tic refers to somites; som**a**tic refers to body wall.)
>
> **Unsegmented mesoderm** is a general, nonspecific term used to indicate embryonic mesoderm that does not form somites. It includes the lateral plate mesoderm (somatic and splanchnic layers) and intermediate mesoderm (nephrotome) connecting somites to the lateral plate.

AXIAL SKELETON

VERTEBRAE AND INTERVERTEBRAL DISKS

The first component of the axial skeleton to appear during development is the notochord, but subsequent development of the vertebral column requires the presence of notochord, neural tube and somites, i.e., sclerotomes. Under the inductive or organizing influence of the notochord, the immediately adjacent portions of the somites (sclerotomes) migrate medially and fuse around the notochord to produce in the midline the segmentally arranged **primary sclerotomes.**

Primary sclerotomes then differentiate into cranial and caudal portions which can be distinguished by marked differences in cellularity. Subsequently, the cranial and caudal halves separate slightly and each dense caudal portion fuses with the cranial portion of the sclerotome below to produce a **secondary** or **definitive sclerotome.**

Secondary sclerotomes will subsequently differentiate into definitive vertebrae and their associated intervertebral disks. The cartilaginous bodies of the vertebrae differentiate from the cell poor areas; the disks from the cell dense areas. The notochord persists throughout the cartilaginous stages of development but disappears during ossification; notochordal remnants persist in the intervertebral disk as the **nucleus pulposus.**

Note: The formation of secondary sclerotomes produces a caudal shift of one-half segment in the definitive vertebral column; this is why intersegmental vessels cross the vertebral body rather than the disk. The half segment shift in the position of the definitive vertebrae assures that the segmental muscles formed by the myotome will operate across an intervertebral articulation rather than arising and inserting on the same bone. The remaining or 'left-over' half sclerotome produced during secondary sclerotome formation and the corresponding segment of the notochord form the **apical ligament of the dens.** The apical ligament extends from the tip of the dens of the axis (epistropheus) to the basioccipital bone and frequently contains a small cartilaginous nodule which is thought to be part of a rudimentary vertebral body.

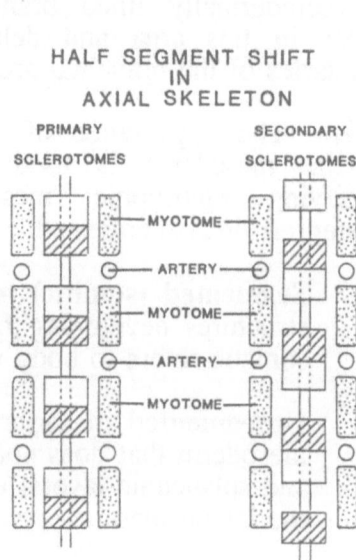

During subsequent development, the cartilaginous vertebral body differentiating from each secondary sclerotome will develop three pairs of processes: **neural arch, transverse** and **costal (rib) processes.**

Neural arch processes grow dorsomedially and fuse across the midline to enclose the developing spinal cord and meninges. Failure of neural arch processes to fuse across the midline on one or two vertebrae, e.g., lower sacral region, is responsible for the minor skeletal defect, **spina bifida occulta.** If the neural arch processes of several adjacent vertebrae are involved, the skeletal defect may allow the meninges and cord to herniate producing the various types of **spina bifida cystica,** e.g., meningocele and meningomyelocele. In myeloschisis (open neural tube) the basic defect occurs much earlier but it is always associated with neural arch defects, i.e., dorsal clefts of the vertebral column (rachischisis).

Transverse processes grow laterally between the dorsal (epimeric) and ventral (hypomeric) musculature of the body wall. Although they are present on all vertebrae, they are the most variable in degree of development.

Costal (rib) processes grow ventrolaterally into the primitive body wall (somatopleura) with other somite derivatives (myotomes and dermatomes); costal processes are usually better developed than transverse processes.

Regional Differentiation of Vertebrae. The serial homology of transverse and costal processes at different trunk levels is obscured and frequently overlooked because of the terms applied to these structures in gross anatomy.

Cervical Vertebrae. The first two cervical vertebrae are highly modified. The atlas has the form of an irregular bony ring without a vertebral body; the axis resembles the other cervical vertebrae but possesses an odontoid process called the dens which represents the missing vertebral body of the atlas. Costal and transverse processes are equally developed on all of the cervical vertebrae and are fused distally to form the cervical transverse process of gross anatomy; the distal tips form the anterior (costal) and posterior (transverse) scalene tubercles. When the costal process is excessively large it produces the readily recognizable cervical rib.

Thoracic Vertebrae. Both costal and transverse processes are readily recognized; the costal (rib) processes reach their maximum development in the thorax.

Lumbar Vertebrae. The transverse processes are reduced to small elevations near the articular facets; the costal processes form the lumbar transverse processes of gross anatomy.

Sacral Vertebrae. The five sacral vertebrae fuse to form the sacrum. The transverse processes are rudimentary as in the lumbar vertebrae; the fused costal processes of the upper three are particularly massive and form the sacral portion of the sacroiliac joint.

Coccygeal Vertebrae. A variable number of coccygeal vertebrae fuse to form the coccyx; they are so rudimentary that only the bodies of four vertebrae are recognizable.

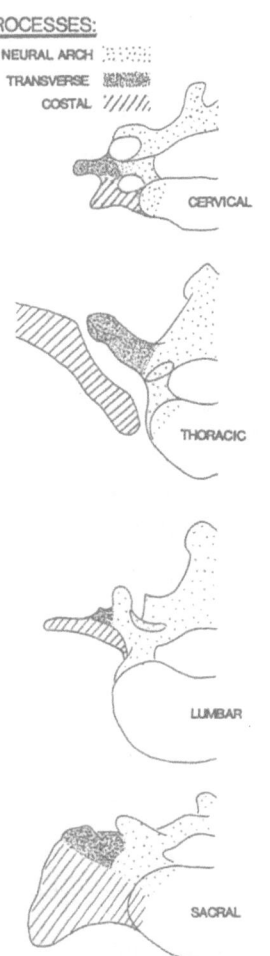

SERIAL HOMOLOGY OF VERTEBRAE

PROCESSES:
NEURAL ARCH
TRANSVERSE
COSTAL

CERVICAL

THORACIC

LUMBAR

SACRAL

SKULL

The skull can be divided into two parts; the **neurocranium**, and the **viscerocranium**. The neurocranium develops from occipital somites and somitomeres and forms the protective case around the brain. The viscerocranium develops from neural crest cells and forms the skeleton of the face. (The development of the viscerocranium will be discussed in Chapter 13: Differentiation of the Branchial Apparatus.)

Neurocranium. The neurocranium can be subdivided into two parts: the **cartilaginous** part which forms the base of the skull; and the **membranous** part which forms the vault of the skull.

Cartilaginous neurocranium. Paraxial mesodermal cells from the somitomeres migrate medially, ventral to the neural tube to participate in forming the cartilaginous neurocranium. In this location they form the parachordal, hypophyseal, trabeculae cranii, and ala orbitalis cartilages. More laterally otic capsules form around the otic vesicles. These cartilages and the occipital sclerotomes fuse and subsequently undergo endochondral ossification to form the base of the skull.

Occipital Sclerotomes. Most of the **occipital bone** of man and higher vertebrates appears to have been formed by the fusion and incorporation of cervical vertebrae into the base of a more primitive and shorter vertebrate skull. The segmental pattern of the four occipital sclerotomes is readily detectable in human embryos but is totally obscured during later development. The boundaries of the **foramen magnum** are formed at least in part by the neural arch processes of the caudalmost segments and it has been suggested that their transverse and/or costal processes contribute to the formation of the occipital condyles. The formation of the caudal part of the skull by what were once cervical vertebrae explains why almost all of the occipital bone develops by endochondral

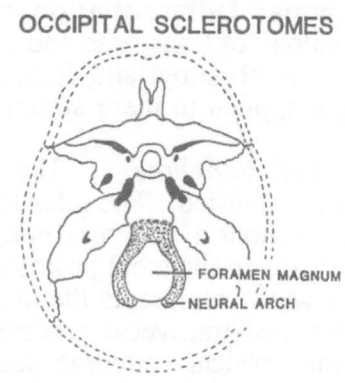

OCCIPITAL SCLEROTOMES

FORAMEN MAGNUM
NEURAL ARCH

ossification like vertebrae whereas other bones of the calvarium develop by intramembranous ossification; only the interparietal portion of the occipital bone develops by intramembranous ossification.

Membranous Neurocranium. Paraxial mesodermal cells from the somitomeres migrate laterally and dorsally to the neural tube and undergo intramembranous ossification to form the membranous neurocranium.

APPENDICULAR SKELETON

The skeletal elements for the limbs and limb girdles develop from lateral plate somatic mesoderm. All of these bones develop by endochondral ossification, with the exception of the clavicle which develops by intramembranous ossification.

DEVELOPMENT OF TRUNK MUSCULATURE

In humans, the musculature of the trunk is derived exclusively from the myotomic portions of somites. Skeletal muscle of myotomic origin is always innervated by large multipolar motor neurons (basal plate) with axons leaving the spinal cord as ventral roots, i.e., **general somatic efferent.** The myotomes are actually responsible for the development of the segmentally arranged motor rootlets of spinal nerves; the association of a presumptive muscle forming mass (myotome) and its motor innervation is established very early in development. The intimate relationship between a myotome and its motor nerve is retained through subsequent stages of migration and differentiation.

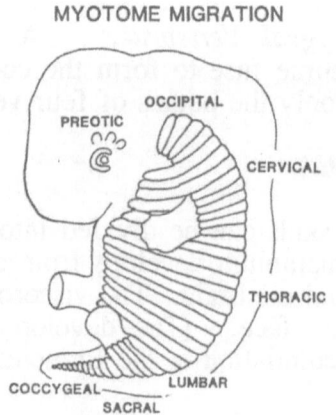

MYOTOME MIGRATION

PREOTIC
OCCIPITAL
CERVICAL
THORACIC
COCCYGEAL
LUMBAR
SACRAL

BODY WALL MUSCULATURE

Dorsal or Epaxial Muscles. As development continues, each myotome divides into an upper or dorsal portion (epimere) which migrates dorsally and medially toward the developing neural arches and transverse processes of the vertebrae. During migration the dorsal portion of the myotome is accompanied by its nerve supply which persists in the adult as the **dorsal primary ramus** (posterior primary division) of a spinal nerve. After reaching their destination along the dorsal aspect of the vertebral column, the dorsal epimeres are subsequently surrounded by an especially dense fascial layer (thoracolumbar and nuchal) and differentiate into the intrinsic muscles of the back (erector spinae complex). The dorsal rami of spinal nerves innervating this group of dorsal muscles retain an unmodified segmental pattern throughout life, i.e., dorsal rami do not form plexi.

Ventral or Hypaxial Muscles. The remaining or ventral portion of each myotome (hypomere) migrates ventrally within the primitive body wall (somatopleura) until it reaches the midline or **linea alba** area of the ventral body wall. During migration the hypomere is accompanied by its nerve supply which persists in the adult as the **ventral primary ramus** (anterior primary division) of a spinal nerve.

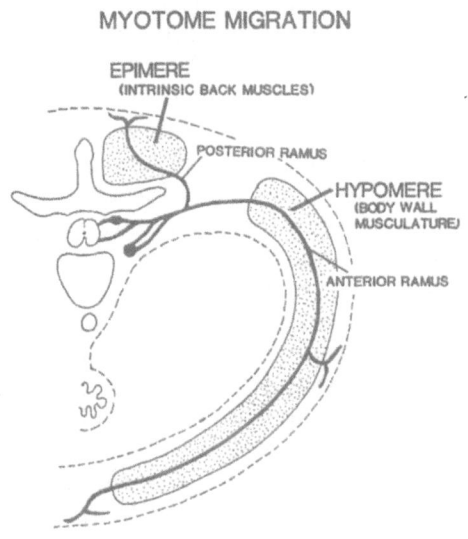

MYOTOME MIGRATION

EPIMERE
(INTRINSIC BACK MUSCLES)

POSTERIOR RAMUS

HYPOMERE
(BODY WALL MUSCULATURE)

ANTERIOR RAMUS

The distribution pattern for the dorsal and ventral rami of typical spinal nerves is produced as the result of myotome migrations. In the adult, the basic segmental pattern of trunk musculature is obvious in the thoracic intercostal muscles, but segmentation is largely obscured in other areas by fusion of adjacent myotomes to form broad sheets (abdominal musculature) or long strap-like muscles (rectus abdominis). Despite these changes (fusions, splittings, etc.), the segmental innervation pattern is retained throughout life.

Note: The **definitive body wall** is formed by the migration of somite derivatives into the primitive somatopleura. The skeletal muscle fibers originate from the somite; the dermis of the skin, connective tissues and fasciae from the dermatomes and somatic layer of the lateral plate. The patterns of muscle formation are determined by the connective tissues into which the myotome migrates.

APPENDICULAR MUSCULATURE

The appendicular musculature is derived exclusively from the **myotomic portions of somites.** Myotome cells migrate into the somatic mesoderm of the limb. The connective tissue (epimysium and perimysium) surrounding the myofibers and adjacent tendons develop from somatic mesoderm. The myogenic cells forming the muscle blastema appear within the developing limb buds as cylindrical masses surrounding the osseous elements of the limb. Very shortly, the cylindrical muscle blastema condenses into two major masses which are oriented along the anterior (ventral) and posterior (dorsal) surfaces of the developing limb. These masses represent the primordia for the primitive flexor (anterior) and extensor (posterior) muscle groups; the primitive muscle masses are separated by lateral and medial septa which will continue to separate the extensor (dorsal) and flexor (ventral) musculature throughout life.

Note: The pattern of limb and girdle musculature formed is determined by the connective tissue (somatic mesoderm) into which the myoblasts migrate.

APPENDICULAR MUSCULATURE AND PLEXUS FORMATION

All appendicular musculature is innervated by branches of **ventral primary rami** from spinal nerves. The ventral primary rami innervating the limb and girdle musculature do not remain segmental, rather they join together at the base of the limb to form **plexi**, e.g., brachial, lumbosacral. The initial segment of the combined rami form the plexus **trunks** which then divide to form anterior and posterior **divisions**. Nerves originating from the anterior and posterior divisions are subsequently distributed to their respective anterior and posterior muscle masses in the limb bud, e.g., in the brachial plexus, the anterior divisions (via the lateral and medial cords) supply nerves for anterior muscles (primitive flexor group) of the upper extremity; the posterior divisions (via the posterior cord) supply nerves for posterior muscles (primitive extensor group) of the upper extremity.

LIMB MUSCULATURE & NERVE PLEXI

ANTERIOR RAMUS

POSTERIOR MUSCLE MASS

ANTERIOR MUSCLE MASS

PRIMITIVE EXTENSORS –ABDUCTORS

MEDIAL SEPTUM — LATERAL SEPTUM

PRIMITIVE FLEXORS –ADDUCTORS

Subsequent changes in the position of the limbs with respect to the trunk (perpendicular during development, parallel in the adult) are largely responsible for the appearance of **adductor** and **abductor** muscle groups operating between the girdle and limb base. Adductor muscles are derived from portions of the primitive anterior (flexor) muscle blastema; flexor and adductor muscles are innervated by nerves arising from the anterior aspect of the plexus. Abductors are derived from portions of the primitive posterior (extensor) muscle blastema; extensor and abductor muscles are innervated by nerves arising from the posterior aspect of the plexus. The relationship between muscle blastemas (anterior and posterior) and divisions (anterior and posterior) of nerve plexi is found in all of the higher vertebrates including man.

CRANIAL MUSCULATURE

Classically, the cranial musculature is considered to be derived from preotic somites, occipital somites, and branchiomeric mesoderm.

Preotic Somites. Classically, the extrinsic occular muscles were considered to be derived from three pairs of preotic somites which are exceedingly transitory structures and appear to contain only the myotomic portion of a typical post-cranial somite. Recent evidence suggests that these skeletal muscles are derived from partially segmented cephalic paraxial mesodermal structures termed somitomeres (see following chart). Myotome-like cells from somitomeres 1-3 and 5 migrate around the developing eye to form the extrinsic occular musculature.

The extrinsic occular musculature is innervated by cranial nerves III (oculomotor), IV (trochlear) and VI (abducens) and differentiate to form the extrinsic muscles of the eye; the arrangement and innervation of eye musculature is unvarying in all vertebrate classes. The motor rootlets of these three cranial nerves arise from large multipolar neurons located in the basal plate of the brain stem but only those of the oculomotor (III) and abducens (VI) exit ventrally; those of the trochlear (IV) grow dorsally within the wall of the mesencephalon, cross and then exit dorsally on the opposite side. This unusual feature of the trochlear nerve (crossing and dorsal exit) is the only known exception to the ventral exit of general somatic efferent fibers and it has never been satisfactorily explained; the same exception is reported to occur in all living vertebrates. It has been suggested by some theoretical morphologists that the muscle mass innervated by the trochlear nerve (superior oblique) may have been originally associated with the midline 'pineal eye' and that as this median visual structure regressed, its musculature assumed a new association with the progressively dominant lateral eyes.

Occipital Somites. Myotomes from the occipital somites migrate anteriorly into the region of the developing oral cavity (stomodaeum and cranial foregut) and subsequently differentiate to form the tongue musculature (intrinsic and extrinsic). During migration, the occipital myotomes are accompanied by their original innervation which is seen in the adult as a series of ventral motor rootlets which combine to form the hypoglossal (XII) nerve. The motor rootlets are derived from large, multipolar motor neurons located in the basal plate of the medulla; the axons exit ventrally like those in ventral roots of all spinal nerves, i.e., they are general somatic efferent.

Branchiomeric Musculature. Classically, the skeletal muscle that develops in association with the branchial apparatus is considered to be derived from branchiomeric mesoderm. **It should be emphasized that recent studies have suggested that branchiomeric musculature, similar to that observed for all other skeletal musculature, is derived from paraxial mesoderm; more specifically from somitomeres and the cranial-most occipital somites.** Paraxial mesodermal cells migrate, along with neural crest cells (ectomesenchyme), lateral and ventral to the pharynx to form the branchial apparatus. During migration the paraxial mesodermal cells are accompanied by their specific cranial nerve.

Note on Skeletal Muscle Innervation. In lower vertebrates, skeletal muscle is regularly derived from both segmented (somites) and unsegmented (lateral plate) mesoderm; the difference in origin is reflected by the exit point of their motor fibers.

Segmented skeletal muscle is innervated by ventrally emerging motor fibers. **Unsegmented** skeletal muscle is innervated by dorsally emerging motor fibers.

The above statements or 'innervation laws' are considered to represent the basic innervation for all chordate skeletal muscle. In higher vertebrates, the amount of skeletal muscle originating from unsegmented or lateral plate mesoderm has been drastically reduced and is thought to persist only in the branchial arches because branchiomeric cranial nerves possess motor fibers which exit dorsally. Dorsal exit of motor fibers explains why mixed cranial nerves (branchiomeric) do not possess dorsal and ventral roots like those of spinal nerves. Dorsal exit also explains why the motor rootlets for the spinal accessory portion of the vagal complex (X-XI) are located above the denticulate ligament while motor rootlets for spinal nerves originating at the same level are below the ligament. Although the developmental significance of dorsal and ventral exit points for motor fibers is not widely recognized by many morphologists, the difference is implied by the nomenclature used to indicate nerve modalities.

General somatic efferent is used to describe motor fibers for skeletal muscle of somite origin; all nerves with this modality (except the trochlear) have motor fibers which exit ventrally.

Special visceral efferent is used to describe motor fibers for skeletal muscle of branchiomeric (unsegmented) origin; all nerves with this modality have motor fibers which exit dorsally, i.e., (V, VII, IX and X-XI).

It must be emphasized that dorsal exit of motor fibers in branchiomeric cranial nerves is NOT an exception to Bell's law; this generalization refers only to nerves possessing dorsal and ventral roots, i.e., spinal nerves.

The following chart describes current thought as to the origin of cranial musculature and its innervation.

CRANIAL NERVE	MESODERMAL ORIGIN	BRANCHIAL ARCH	FUNCT. COMP.	MUSCLES
oculomotor (III)	SO 1,2 (preotic somite)		GSE	superior, medial and ventral recti
trochlear (IV)	SO 3 (preotic somite)		GSE	superior oblique
mandibular branch of trigeminal (V₃)	SO 4	1	SVE	muscles of mastication and jaw-closing muscles
abducens (VI)	SO 5		GSE	lateral rectus
facial (VII)	SO 6	2	SVE	muscles of facial expression and jaw opening muscles
glossopharyngeal (IX)	SO 7	3	SVE	stylopharyngeus
superior laryngeal of vagus (X)	SI 1,2	4	SVE	pharyngeal, cricothyroid
inferior laryngeal of vagus (X)	SI 1,2	6	SVE	laryngeal
spinal accessory (XI)	SI 1,2	caudal to branchial apparatus	SVE	trapezius, sternocleidomastoid
hypoglossal (XII)	SI 2-4		GSE	tongue

SO - somitomere
SI - occipital somite

Note: The pattern of musculature formed in association with the branchial apparatus is determined by the connective tissue (ectomesenchyme) into which the myoblasts migrate.

DEVELOPMENTAL DEFECTS

Failure of somites to appear during early development will produce a shortened body axis accompanied by a reduction in the number of spinal nerves. Conversely, extra somites produce an elongated body axis accompanied by an increase in spinal nerves. On rare occasions, individuals are born with severe scoliosis and upon examination are found to possess one or more hemivertebrae (half vertebrae); the developmental basis for forming half vertebrae can result from asymmetrical:

1. somite formation, i.e., somites do not form in pairs.
2. formation of primary and secondary sclerotomes.
3. formation of the **bilateral** ossifications centers for the cartilaginous model of the vertebral body.

Failure of a somite to appear on one side would be reflected by absence of the corresponding spinal nerve, i.e, a myotome was never present to induce nerve formation. Later regression or degeneration of a normally formed somite may produce skeletal (sclerotomic) or muscle (myotomic) defects without reducing the number of spinal nerves.

Major muscle defects are most commonly those related to failure or incomplete migration of the hypomere within the primitive body wall. In these cases, the body wall remains thin and transparent because the somatopleura lacks the migratory somite derivatives; normal differentiation of the integumentary system (epidermis as well as dermis) does not occur in the absence of underlying muscle. Defects in the anterior body wall with direct exposure of the viscera (thoracoschisis, gastroschisis, exstrophy of the bladder) is often explained by failure of the lateral body folds to fuse in the midline. Such explanations are misleading because the body wall in man and other mammals is always a complete (except at the umbilicus) but delicate membrane formed by the somatopleura. These defects are almost invariably associated with failure or incomplete migration of somite derivatives within the primitive body wall; rupture of the persisting somatopleura during labor is responsible for external exposure of the viscera.

QUESTIONS: Chapter 10 - Musculoskeletal System

1.   The embryonic coelom or body cavity forms within the:
    A.   paraxial mesoderm
    B.   lateral plate mesoderm
    C.   branchiomeric mesoderm
    D.   somatic layer of mesoderm
    E.   splanchnic layer of mesoderm

2.   The sclerotomic portion of somites are known to make contributions to all of the following **EXCEPT** the:
    A.   secondary sclerotomes
    B.   vertebrae
    C.   sacrum
    D.   humerus
    F.   occipital bone

3.   **ALL** of the skeletal muscle found in the developing human is derived from:
    A.   neural crest mesenchyme (ectomesenchyme)
    B.   paraxial mesoderm
    C.   lateral plate mesoderm
    D.   somatic layer of mesoderm
    E.   splanchnic layer of mesoderm

4.   Skeletal muscles which develop in association with the branchial apparatus receive their motor innervation via nerves possessing the modality:
    A.   general somatic efferent.
    B.   general visceral efferent.
    C.   special somatic afferent.
    D.   special visceral efferent.
    E.   none of the above.

5.   The viscerocranium is derived from:
    A.   cephalic paraxial mesoderm.
    B.   neural crest cells.
    C.   lateral plate mesoderm.
    D.   secondary sclerotome.
    E.   pharyngeal endoderm.

6.   The formation of an extra pair of somites at the thoracic level would be expected to result in all of the following structures duplicated **EXCEPT**:
    A.   intercostal nerves
    B.   intercostal arteries
    C.   intervertebral disks
    D.   vertebrae
    E.   digits

Answers: 1=B; 2=D; 3=B; 4=D; 5=B; 6=E

CHAPTER 11: INTEGUMENTARY SYSTEM

The skin or integument receives major contributions from two germ layers: ectoderm and mesoderm. The **epidermis** is derived from the ectoderm covering the outer surface of the embryo; the **dermis** or corium is derived from mesoderm. The connective tissue forming the dermis is usually considered to be derived from the dermatomic portion of the somite with some contributions from the somatic layer of the primitive body wall (somatopleura).

Normal differentiation of the epidermis and general integumentary structures (hair and glands) appears to occur only in the presence of underlying skeletal muscle derived from myotomes or branchiomeric mesenchyme. In the trunk at least, normal development of the skin does not occur when the underlying musculature is missing.

GENERAL INTEGUMENTARY COVERING

Epidermis. Initially, the ectodermal epithelium covering the embryo is composed of a simple cuboidal epithelium. Subsequent proliferation of the ectodermal epithelium produces a second layer of cells which is referred to as the **periderm** or epitrichium. The periderm is a transitory layer and will be lost during later stages of differentiation; the deeper layer of cuboidal cells will persist throughout life as the **basal cell layer** (stratum basale) of the epidermis. As the basal cells continue to proliferate, an intermediate layer of cells begins to accumulate below the periderm; this third layer contains the **prickle cells** or developing **keratinocytes** of the stratum spinosum, i.e., Malpighian layer. A short time later, the superficial cells will begin to mature (keratinize) and slough into the amniotic fluid. Loss of the periderm or epitrichium appears to coincide with the eruption of developing hair shafts.

Vernix caseosa is a white fatty secretion product produced by the fetal sebaceous glands; it is particularly thick over the scalp, back and skin creases around joints. It is thought to protect the fetus from maceration by amniotic fluid during the later stages of development but it may represent nothing more than the gradual accumulation of normal secretory products and desquamating cells on the surface of an integument in a protected environment, i.e., in utero.

Pigment Cells. Neural crest cells appear in the deepest layer of the developing epidermis (basal cell layer) during the first month of fetal life and subsequently complete their differentiation into the dendritic or pigment producing cells of the skin, i.e., **melanocytes**. Localized accumulations of cutaneous neural crest cells (presumptive melanocytes) are responsible for the formation of 'moles' or pigmented nevi.

Developmental Defects. Most of the severe developmental defects affecting the general integumentary covering of the body wall are related to migration failures of somite derivatives. Pigmentation (moles) and vascular (angiomas) malformations are minor development anomalies and can be found in almost any body area; most are small and insignificant. Occasionally, however, these malformations may be quite large and are disfiguring when present on the face, scalp or neck, e.g., deeply pigmented and elevated nevi, port wine stain.

EPIDERMIS

ECTODERM

MESENCHYME

PERIDERM

BASAL CELL LAYER

S. INTERMEDIUM

MIGRATING NEURAL CREST CELLS

EPIDERMIS

MELANOCYTES

SPECIALIZED INTEGUMENTARY STRUCTURES

Note: All of the specialized integumentary structures (glands, hair, teeth, nails) are formed by the same basic developmental process, i.e., proliferation of the basal cell layer of the epidermis into the underlying mesenchyme.

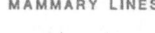

MAMMARY GLANDS

Mammary glands are the most characteristic feature of mammals and are the first specialized integumentary structures to appear. The ectodermal band forming the **mammary ridge** or line appears on the anterior body wall during the sixth week of embryonic life and extends caudally from the axillary to the inguinal region. In humans, mammae are restricted to the pectoral region and as a consequence, portions of the mammary line cranial and caudal to this area regress. In the pectoral region, 16-24 solid cords of epithelial cells appear within a small circumscribed (nipple) area and continue to grow and branch within the adjacent mesenchyme. These epithelial cords are the primordia for the 16-24 **lactiferous ducts** and **sinuses** found in the adult. Although canalization occurs during the latter half of pregnancy, the mammary gland of the newborn consists primarily of proximal ducts with a few rudimentary acini. Ducts and acini are comprised of inner and outer cell layers; the inner layer will persist to form the epithelium for the definitive ducts and acini; the outer layer of

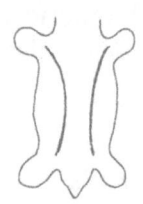

cells will ultimately differentiate into the discontinuous layer of **myoepithelial cells**. Witch's milk, a secretory product of the newborn mammae, is thought to be produced as a result of high levels of fetal steroids (estrogen and progesterone) and placental lactogen. The rudimentary acini regress and secretion ceases as hormone levels decline following parturition.

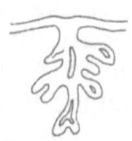

Developmental Defects. **Polythelia** or extra nipples is very common and may occur as elevated or pedunculated pigmented 'moles' anywhere along the mammary line, i.e., axilla to medial surface of the thigh. **Polymastia** or extra mammary glands is very rare but they have been reported from the axilla to the medial surface of the thigh. **Amastia** or complete absence of a mammary gland on one or both sides is so rare that the defect is almost nonexistent.

TEETH

Although they are not exclusively mammalian characteristics, teeth are the second specialized integumentary structures to appear. The **dental laminae** for the upper and lower jaws appear in the stomodeal (ectodermal) portion of the oral cavity during the seventh week of development; the two laminae will subsequently form enamel organs for all of the deciduous (20) and permanent (32) teeth. The **ameloblasts** of the ectodermally derived enamel organ will secrete only the enamel covering for the crown of the tooth. **Odontoblasts** originating from the neural crest mesenchyme of the dental papilla will form the dentin for all remaining parts of the tooth, i.e., dentin supporting the enamel and forming the roots of the tooth. Although the enamel organs for the 32 permanent teeth begin to appear during fetal life, their formation is not complete at birth. The enamel organs for the last permanent molars (wisdom teeth) develop at about the age of five years; this is one of the reasons that tetracyclines, which localize in mineralizing tissues, should be used with caution in pregnant women, infants and young children. Exposure to high fluoride levels during childhood may produce discoloration and/or irregularities in the enamel of the permanent dentition.

Note: The type of tooth formed (incisor, molar, etc.,) is determined by the neural crest cells located under the dental laminae. When neural crest mesenchyme from a molar-forming area is transplanted to the premaxillary area, the overlying ectoderm responds by producing an enamel organ for a molar rather than one for the incisor normally developing in this area. Even more spectacular are the transplantation experiments in which dental neural crest cells from mammals are transplanted to birds; although birds have not developed teeth for millions of years, the avian ectoderm responds by producing an enamel organ appropriate for the transplanted mammalian neural crest cells.

Developmental Defects. Some abnormalities in tooth morphology and number are familial traits; most if not all, appear to be inherited as autosomal dominants. A reduction or increase in the number of enamel organs produced by the dental laminae (deciduous or permanent) will be reflected at the time of tooth eruption by missing or extra teeth.

HAIR

SWEAT GLAND

Although hairs, like mammae, are characteristic features of mammals, they appear relatively late in development; hair follicles first appear on the head and face during the third month. The hair produced by these follicles is very fine and dense but this **lanugo hair** is normally shed before or shortly after birth. Lanugo hair is replaced by coarse and less dense hair produced from later developing follicles.

SEBACEOUS GLANDS

HAIR FOLLICLE

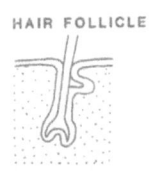

Primordia for sebaceous glands usually develop from the epithelial cells of hair follicles and are, therefore, somewhat later to appear (4-5 months) than the other integumentary structures. The central cells of the gland primordia undergo fatty degeneration of the **holocrine** type to form the fatty component of the vernix caseosa.

ENAMEL ORGAN

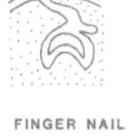

SWEAT GLANDS

FINGER NAIL

The unbranched epithelial cords forming the sweat gland primordia appear on the palmar and plantar surfaces of the extremities during the third month and canalize a short time later. After canalization, the coiled, unbranched epithelial tube is composed of an inner and outer layer of cells. The outer layer will subsequently become discontinuous and ultimately differentiate into myoepithelial cells; the inner layer will persist as the secretory and ductal epithelial cells.

NAILS

The plate-like epithelial folds forming the primordia for nails appear near the tips of the digits during the third month. After formation, the nail folds appear to migrate to a more proximal location on the dorsal aspect of the digits; dorsal migration is thought to explain why the nails and adjacent skin on the dorsal surface of digits are innervated by nerves derived from ventral cutaneous nerves supplying the palmar and plantar surfaces. Nails grow slowly during fetal life and reach the tip of the digits about the time of parturition.

Note: The major papillary ridges responsible for fingerprints (dermatoglyphs) appear on the digits about the middle of fetal life.

EYELIDS

The eyelids develop as folds of skin above and below the eyes; the folds fuse during the third month and do not reopen until the seventh month. Epithelial cords forming the primordia for the lacrimal gland develop in the lateral part of superior palpebral fold; the lacrimal gland is completely formed at birth but it is small and does not become fully functional for several weeks. Development of the specialized palpebral hair (cilia or lashes), sebaceous (Zeis and Meibomian) and sweat (Moll) glands is comparable to that occurring in other integumentary areas.

QUESTIONS: Chapter 11 - Integumentary System

1. The first recognizable layer of the epidermis to appear during early embryogenesis is the:
    A. periderm
    B. vernix caseosa
    C. keratinocyte layer (Malpighian layer)
    D. basal cell layer
    E. none of the above

2. Which of the following integumentary cells is **NOT** derived from the surfacing ectoderm?
    A. keratinocyte
    B. ameloblast
    C. melanocyte
    D. peridermal cell
    E. myoepithelial cell

3. Surface ectoderm forming the dental laminae will give rise to:
    A. dentin
    B. dental papilla
    C. enamel
    D. odontoblasts
    E. none of the above

4. In terms of total dentition (deciduous and permanent), the functional life span of the dental lamina in humans is approximately:
    A. one year
    B. three years
    C. five years
    D. eighteen years
    E. twenty-one years

5. The presence of an extra mammary gland (polymastia) in the inguinal region can best be explained by:
    A. failure of myotomes to invade the primitive body wall
    B. caudal displacement and fusion of the mammary lines
    C. failure of the mammary line to regress at caudal levels
    D. overgrowth with caudal extension of the mammary line
    E. incomplete migration of neural crest cells

6. Epithelial invasion of the underlying mesoderm occurs during formation of:
    A. enamel organs
    B. hair follicles
    C. finger nails
    D. sebaceous glands
    E. all of the above

Answers: 1=D; 2=C; 3=C; 4=C; 5=C; 6=E

CHAPTER 12: ORAL CAVITY AND DEVELOPMENT OF THE BRANCHIAL APPARATUS

In the trilaminar embryo, the area of the future oral cavity is indicated by the oropharyngeal membrane; this structure is located in the midline between the cephalic end of the notochord and the developing cardiogenic area. The oropharyngeal membrane is a thin, circular area comprised of ectodermal and endodermal epithelium; the apposed epithelial layers in this area are firmly adherent and thus prevent invasion and vascularization by the adjacent mesoderm. Subsequent degeneration of the avascular oropharyngeal membrane is responsible for producing the oral opening. During head fold formation, the oropharyngeal membrane and cardiogenic area, which are cranial to the notochord, are folded ventrally and caudally to form the floor of the foregut and the anterior body wall above the umbilicus. Head fold formation is especially important because it moves the future oral cavity to its definitive location on the anterior surface of the body and because it establishes the permanent anatomical relationships between the developing heart, pharyngeal foregut and their associated coelomic spaces, i.e., pericardial and pleural cavities.

PRIMITIVE ORAL CAVITY

While head fold formation is in progress, proliferation of embryonic mesenchyme around the circumference of the oropharyngeal membrane produces a pit-like depression lined with ectoderm which is referred to as the **stomodeum** or **primitive oral cavity**. At this stage of development, the oropharyngeal membrane is intact within the stomodeal depression and separates the lumen of the primitive oral cavity (stomodeum) from the lumen of the pharyngeal foregut.   Shortly   before   the   oropharyngeal   membrane degenerates, a midline epithelial outgrowth from the floor of the foregut produces the endodermal primordium (thyroglossal duct) for the **thyroid gland**; a short time later, a comparable epithelial outgrowth from the roof of the stomodeum produces the ectodermal primordium (Rathke's pouch) for the anterior lobe   of   the   pituitary   gland,   i.e.,   **adenohypophysis**. Immediately after the appearance of the thyroid and pituitary primordia, the avascular oropharyngeal membrane degenerates and continuity between the lumen of the primitive oral cavity and that of the pharyngeal foregut is finally established.

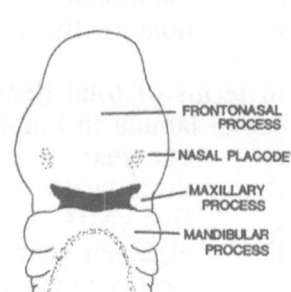

PRIMITIVE ORAL CAVITY

- FRONTONASAL PROCESS
- NASAL PLACODE
- MAXILLARY PROCESS
- MANDIBULAR PROCESS

Degeneration of the oropharyngeal membrane does not leave distinctive landmarks in the oral mucosa to indicate the stomodeum-foregut junction, but its approximate location in the adult is slightly rostral to the **foramen cecum** (origin of thyroid) on the base of the tongue. The caudal limits of the stomodeal ectoderm can be approximated from the last molar teeth since their enamel was formed by the ectodermally derived ameloblasts.

DEFINITIVE ORAL CAVITY

The palate (hard and soft), which forms during differentiation of the branchial apparatus, divides the primitive oral cavity into dorsal (respiratory) and ventral (digestive) passages.

Dorsally, the respiratory part of the primitive oral cavity forms almost all of the paired **nasal cavities**; the adjacent **nasopharynx** is formed by the dorsal wall of the pharyngeal foregut.

Ventrally, the digestive part of the primitive oral cavity forms the anterior two-thirds of the oral cavity and tongue; the posterior one-third of these structures is formed by the adjacent **oropharynx** or ventral wall of the foregut.

Note: The palate is an exclusively stomodeal structure and it separates the respiratory and digestive passages at the oral levels only. However, since the respiratory and digestive passages must cross at the pharyngeal levels, the foregut must remain undivided to provide this common respiratory-digestive channel; the naso- and oropharynx are formed, respectively, by the dorsal and ventral walls of this common channel, i.e., the pharyngeal foregut.

Tongue development will be covered at the end of the following chapter because, in addition to its contributions from the occipital somites, stomodeum and pharyngeal foregut, it also receives contributions from the branchial apparatus.

BRANCHIAL APPARATUS

Almost all of the structures found in the head and neck are associated with the development and differentiation of a series of structural complexes (branchial arches) which are referred to collectively as the **branchial apparatus.** It must be emphasized, however, that the serial or repeating structure of branchial arches is found in the lateral wall of the pharyngeal foregut and is unrelated to somite formation. It is also important to remember that almost all of the mesenchyme found in the cephalic region of the embryo appears after head fold formation. As a consequence of its late appearance, this mesenchyme is not split into somatic and splanchnic layers by coelom formation and persists as a single layer which is referred to as the **branchiomeric mesenchyme.** A short time later, the walls of the pharyngeal foregut are characterized by the appearance of the branchial arches and it is for this reason that the mesenchyme in this area is referred to as **branchiomeric.**

BRANCHIOMERIC MESENCHYME

Most of the branchiomeric mesenchyme originates from the cephalic neural crest and will eventually differentiate into many of the skeletal elements (bone and cartilage) and other connective tissues (areolar, dense, etc.,) found in the head and neck. The origin of the myogenic portion of the branchiomeric mesenchyme is controversial (paraxial versus lateral plate mesoderm) but it will subsequently form all of the skeletal muscle found in the head and pharynx except those originating from the occipital and preotic somites, i.e., tongue and eye musculature.

BRANCHIAL ARCH FORMATION

The first and most prominent pair of branchial arches develops from localized accumulations of branchiomeric mesenchyme around the periphery of the oropharyngeal membrane. The first arch (mandibular) and its derivatives will ultimately form the upper and lower jaws of the definitive oral cavity and it is the accumulation of branchiomeric mesenchymal cells for the first arch that produces the pit-like stomodeal depression of the primitive oral cavity.

As post-mandibular arches continue to form in the lateral wall of the pharyngeal foregut, they are separated from adjacent arches by the formation of external **branchial grooves** and internal **pharyngeal pouches.** The epithelial components of the branchial grooves (ectoderm) and pharyngeal pouches (endoderm) approach each other through the pharyngeal body wall and come into direct apposition to form the **branchial membranes.** In lower vertebrates, the avascular branchial membranes soon degenerate to form functional gill-slits, but in the higher vertebrates, including man, branchial membrane degeneration does not occur because the epithelial layers are quickly re-separated and vascularized by the adjacent branchiomeric mesenchyme.

When formation of the branchial arches is complete, the maxillary and mandibular portions of the first arch form the lateral and inferior boundaries of the primitive oral cavity (stomodeum); arches caudal to the first or mandibular arch form the lateral and inferior walls of the pharyngeal foregut.

Note: The number of branchial arches formed during human development is variously reported by different embryologists to be either five or six; the inconsistency in arch number arises from the basis used for numbering. In human embryos, five complete arches are formed; the sixth pair is often uncounted because its caudal boundaries are not delineated by grooves and pouches, i.e., the caudal part of the 'incomplete' sixth arch is continuous with the post-branchial arch body wall. The sixth arch is always included in the numbering systems used throughout this review.

AORTIC ARCHES

It should be noted that at some time during their early formative stages, each branchial arch becomes vascularized by vessels originating from the ventral (truncus arteriosus) and dorsal aortae. These vessels are the paired **aortic arches**; all six pairs are not present at any one time during development. The contributions of the aortic arches to the definitive arterial vasculature will be presented with cardiovascular development.

BRANCHIOMERIC NERVES

During its formation, the first branchial arch becomes associated with the developing trigeminal nerve; the trigeminal nerve will eventually supply the major afferent (sensory) and efferent (motor) innervation for all first arch derivatives. As successive branchial arches appear, each will form a comparable association with one of the other branchiomeric nerves. The association between a branchial arch and its branchiomeric nerve is the same in all vertebrates, i.e., the first arch is always innervated by the trigeminal (V); the second arch is always innervated by the facial (VII); the third arch is always innervated by the glossopharyngeal (IX); the fourth and all arches caudal to the fourth are always innervated by the vagal complex (X-XI).

Note: The accessory nerve (XI) is a partially detached motor branch of the vagus and supplies innervation for muscle derivatives of the sixth arch; the sensory components for sixth arch derivatives have remained with the vagus.

QUESTIONS: Chapter 12 - Oral Cavity and Development of the Branchial Apparatus

1. Which of the following branchial arch/cranial nerve relationships is **INCORRECT?**
    A. arch 6 - accessory portion of the vagal complex (X and XI)
    B. arch 4 - vagal portion of the vagal complex (X and XI)
    C. arch 3 - hypoglossal
    D. arch 2 - facial
    E. arch 1 - trigeminal

2. Structures originating wholly or in part from stomodeal ectoderm include:
    A. teeth
    B. nasal mucosa
    C. oral mucosa
    D. adenohypophysis
    E. all of the above

3. Choose the **CORRECT** statement concerning branchiomeric mesenchyme.
    A. Most of it develops from cephalic neural crest cells.
    B. It develops after coelom and head fold formation.
    C. It is innervated by nerves possessing special visceral efferent fibers.
    D. It forms skeletal muscle which is histologically identical to that formed from myotomes.
    E. All of the above statements are true.

4. A typical branchial arch contains:
    A. a cranial nerve
    B. branchiomeric mesenchyme
    C. an aortic arch
    D. a skeletal element
    E. all of the above

5. Immediately following its formation, the superior boundary of the stomodeal depression or oral cavity is formed by the:
    A. maxillary processes of the first branchial arch
    B. mandibular processes of the first branchial arch
    C. frontonasal prominence
    D. lateral nasal prominence
    E. hyoid arch

6. The oropharyngeal membrane:
    A. separates stomodeum and pharynx
    B. contains an outer layer composed of ectoderm
    C. is moved ventrally and caudally during head fold formation
    D. is located just rostral to the foramen cecum in the embryo
    E. all of the following

Answers: 1=C; 2=E; 3=E; 4=E; 5=C; 6=E

CHAPTER 13: DIFFERENTIATION OF THE BRANCHIAL APPARATUS

Branchial arches are structural complexes containing cells and tissues of diverse embryological origin. Each arch complex consists of a central core of branchiomeric mesenchyme containing a large arterial vessel (aortic arch) and a nerve; the central core is enclosed by an epithelial layer derived in part from body wall ectoderm and in part from foregut endoderm.

The boundaries of the first five arches are delineated by **branchial grooves** and **pharyngeal pouches** which, like the arches, are numbered; both grooves and pouches are located caudal to the arch with the corresponding number. The caudal limits of the sixth arch are not indicated by the presence of grooves and pouches and as a consequent it is directly continuous with the post-branchial body wall; the 'incomplete' sixth arch does contain, however, all of the components found in the other five arches.

BRANCHIOMERIC MESENCHYME

During differentiation, the neural crest component of branchiomeric mesenchyme will form all **skeletal elements** (bone, cartilage, ligaments) appearing within that arch; the myogenic component will form all of the **skeletal muscle** found in the head except those formed from the occipital and preotic somites (tongue and eye musculature). As the branchiomeric skeletal muscles differentiate, they will receive their **special visceral efferent** innervation from the nerve associated with the arch of origin.

BRANCHIAL ARCH EPITHELIUM

Branchial arches develop in a region of the body lacking a coelomic space and as a consequence, each arch represents a column of combined body and gut wall. The external or ectodermal portion is comparable to the somatopleura found elsewhere and will eventually form **cutaneous areas** in the integument of the head; conversely, the internal or endodermal portion is comparable to splanchnopleura and will eventually form **mucosal areas** in the oropharyngeal cavity. The contributions made to cutaneous and mucosal surfaces by individual arches are extremely variable in size. **General somatic afferent** (skin) and **general visceral afferent** (mucosa) fibers for ectodermal and endodermal epithelial surfaces originate from the nerve of the contributing arch; however, **special visceral afferent** fibers for taste buds in one area are always derived from the nerve located in the arch behind it. Separate origins for general and special fibers are responsible for producing the unusual overlapping innervation pattern found in the oropharyngeal mucosa and explains why the anterior two-thirds of the tongue receives its general afferent innervation from the trigeminal (lingual branch of V3) while taste buds in the-same area receive their special afferent fibers from the chorda tympani branch of the facial nerve.

FATE OF THE BRANCHIOMERIC MESENCHYME

BRANCHIAL ARCH I

Skeletal Element. Meckel's cartilage is the skeletal element of the first arch. The dorsal or upper end undergoes endochondral ossification to form the **malleus** and **incus** bones of the middle ear; the intermediate portion regresses leaving the fibrous **anterior malleolar** and **sphenomandibular ligaments** between the ear ossicles and the lower jaw. The ventral or lower portion eventually disappears without making significant contributions to the lower jaw. **Note:** The mandible and maxillae develop independently by intramembranous ossification from mesenchymal cells located within the mandibular and maxillary processes of the first arch.

Muscles.   The musculature originating from the first arch receives its special visceral efferent innervation from the mandibular (V_3) division of the trigeminal nerve. Although most of this musculature becomes associated with the mandible to form the **muscles of mastication**, a small portion retains its association with the malleus (Meckel's cartilage) to form the **tensor tympani muscle.**

BRANCHIAL ARCH II

Skeletal Element.   Reichert's cartilage is the skeletal element of the second arch. The dorsal or upper end undergoes endochondral ossification to form the **stapes and styloid process;** the intermediate portion forms the **stylohyoid ligament** extending to the lesser cornu of the hyoid; the lower end undergoes endochondral ossification to form the **lesser cornu** and **upper half of the hyoid.**

Muscles.   The musculature originating from the second arch receives its special visceral efferent innervation from the facial nerve (VII); the myoblasts migrate in the superficial fascia throughout the head, neck and upper thorax to form the muscles of facial expression. A small dorsal portion retains its association with the stapes (Reichert's cartilage) to form the **stapedius** muscle. Two other muscles form, the stylohyoid and posterior belly of the digastric, which extend from the styloid process to the hyoid bone.

BRANCHIAL ARCH III

Skeletal Element.   The cartilaginous element disappears dorsally; the ventral portion undergoes endochondral ossification to form the **greater cornu** and **lower half of the hyoid.**

Muscles.   The **stylopharyngeus** is the only specifically named muscle receiving special visceral efferent fibers from the glossopharyngeal nerve (IX). There is some evidence to indicate that it may also make some contributions to the upper portion of the pharyngeal constrictors but the pharyngeal branch of IX is usually considered to contain only afferent fibers.

BRANCHIAL ARCHES IV, V and VI

Skeletal Elements.   The cartilaginous supporting elements of arches four, five and six are rudimentary; all are thought to contribute to the formation of the laryngeal cartilages (thyroid, cricoid, arytenoid).

Muscles.   Special visceral efferent fibers from the vagal complex (X-XI) supply all of the pharyngeal, laryngeal and appendicular muscles originating from arches four, five and six.

The fourth arch nerve is the **superior laryngeal branch** of the vagus; it supplies musculature of both the larynx (cricothyroid) and pharynx (upper constrictors).

The fifth arch nerve is a **pharyngeal branch** of the vagus; it supplies musculature for the pharynx only (intermediate constrictors).

The sixth arch nerve is the **accessory** part of the vagus; it supplies musculature for the larynx, pharynx and the upper appendage.   The appendicular musculature (trapezius and sternocleidomastoid) is supplied by the accessory nerve directly, but the pharyngeal (lower constrictors and upper esophageal) and laryngeal musculature (except cricothyroid) are supplied by accessory fibers in the vagus, i.e., the inferior or recurrent laryngeal nerve.

FATE OF THE PHARYNGEAL POUCHES

The branchial arches are separated internally by the pharyngeal pouches and, as a consequence, the cranial and caudal boundaries of each pouch are formed by the endodermal epithelium of the adjacent arches. The pouches are located caudal to the arches with the corresponding number.

Note: The endodermal epithelium of both the arch and pouch is presumptive oropharyngeal mucosa; these endodermal mucosal areas will receive their general visceral afferent innervation from the branchiomeric nerve associated with that arch. However, the same mucosal area will always receive its special visceral afferent (taste) and autonomic (general visceral efferent) fibers from the nerve associated with the adjacent lower arch. In humans, the chorda tympani is the only easily recognizable example of this overlapping innervation pattern.

PHARYNGEAL POUCH I

The first pouch forms the **pharyngotympanic tube (Eustachian), cavity** of the middle ear and inner mucosal layer of the **tympanic membrane**. Dorsal expansion of the first pouch surrounds the bones developing from the dorsal ends of Meckel's (malleus and incus) and Reichert's (stapes) cartilages and establishes the definitive relationship of ear ossicles traversing the cavity of the middle ear. Dorsal expansion of the first pouch also explains the definitive location of the chorda tympani nerve in the tympanic membrane. Because the boundaries of the first pouch are formed by the endodermal epithelium of the first and second arches, the general visceral afferent innervation for the oropharyngeal mucosa in this area is derived from the adjacent trigeminal and facial nerves.

BRANCHIAL APPARATUS

STOMODEAL DEPRESSION
ORAL MEMBRANE
POUCHES
GROOVES
1 1
2 2
3 3
4 4
5 5

ECTODERM OF BODY WALL ————
ENDODERM OF FOREGUT - - - - - - -

PHARYNGEAL POUCH II

The second pouch forms the epithelium and crypts of the palatine tonsil; the lymphocytes will migrate into this area later. The general visceral afferent innervation for the oropharyngeal mucosa in this area is derived from the adjacent facial and glossopharyngeal nerves.

PHARYNGEAL POUCH III

Pouch three forms the **inferior parathyroids** and the endodermal primordium for the **epithelial reticulum** of the definitive thymus; lymphocytes begin to invade the thymic epithelial cords at about nine weeks. Developmental defects involving the third pouch may result in thymic aplasia or hypoplasia with or without involvement of the inferior parathyroids. DiGeorge syndrome is characterized by thymic agenesis with impaired cell mediated immunity and with hypoparathyroidism and tetany; complete absence of parathyroids with tetany suggests a more extensive defect involving the fourth pouch. The third pouch loses its epithelial connection with the pharynx but the mucosal areas of the associated third and fourth arches receive their general visceral afferent innervation from the glossopharyngeal and vagus nerves.

PHARYNGEAL POUCH IV

Pouch number four forms the **superior parathyroids** and contributes to the formation of the ultimobranchial body; the pharyngeal mucosa in this area will receive its general visceral afferent innervation from separate but adjacent pharyngeal branches of the vagus.

PHARYNGEAL POUCH V

The fifth and last pouch is usually considered to form the ultimobranchial body; it probably receives some contributions from the fourth pouch. During subsequent development this structure becomes incorporated into the developing thyroid and for some time it was considered to be the source of the parafollicular or calcitonin-producing C-cells. Recent evidence indicates that the C-cells originate from neural crest, become associated with the ultimobranchial body and subsequently differentiate into the parafollicular C-cells of the thyroid. The significance of their association with the ultimobranchial body is not known. The pharyngeal mucosa in the areas of the fifth pouch receives its general visceral afferent innervation from separate but adjacent pharyngeal branches of the vagus (the accessory has no afferent component of its own).

FATE OF THE BRANCHIAL GROOVES

The ectodermal epithelium of the stomodeum, branchial arches and grooves is the presumptive integumentary epithelium for the future oral cavity and skin. All of the ectodermal epithelial areas will receive their general somatic afferent innervation from the nerves of the arches involved, i.e., the stomodeal portions of the nasal cavities and anterior oral cavity receive these fibers from the maxillary (V_2) and mandibular (V_3) divisions of the trigeminal. All nerves (cranial and spinal) supplying ectodermal or integumentary areas possess this modality.

BRANCHIAL GROOVE I

The first branchial groove persists as the **external auditory canal** and its contribution to the branchial membrane persists to form the outer layer of the **tympanic membrane**. The general somatic afferent innervation for this area is derived from the nerves of the adjacent arches, i.e., trigeminal and facial.

BRANCHIAL GROOVES II, III, IV and V

All grooves caudal to the first are obliterated by mesodermal infilling. Each arch has some cutaneous representation but only that of the fourth arch is associated with a specifically named nerve, i.e., the auricular branch of the vagus.

It is sometimes implied that the caudal arches are overgrown and the cervical sinus obliterated by caudal growth of the second arch. The caudal growth is more apparent than real and is caused by myoblasts migrating from the region of the second arch to form the cervical and thoracic portions of the platysma. If the entire arch grew caudally, the cutaneous area covering the platysma would receive its general somatic afferent innervation from the facial rather than from cervical nerves two, three and four. Entrapped epithelial remnants of the branchial grooves and cervical sinus may persist to form branchial cysts or sinuses during later life; both are usually located under or anterior to the sternocleidomastoid.

FORMATION OF THE TONGUE

The definitive tongue and oral cavity originate from the stomodeum and pharyngeal foregut; the foramen cecum indicates the approximate dividing line between the ectodermal and endodermal contributions.

The first indications of tongue development occur in the stomodeum with the appearance of the **tuberculum impar** and the **lateral lingual swellings**; this is followed by the appearance of the **copula** (second arch area) and **hypobranchial eminence** (third and fourth arch areas). The anterior two-thirds or body of the tongue is formed by growth and fusion of the lateral lingual swellings; a contribution from the tuberculum impar cannot be identified. In the pharyngeal area, the cranial part of the branchial eminence (third arch) appears to overgrow the copula and eventually fuses with the stomodeal contributions to complete the base of the tongue; the **sulcus terminalis** indicates the site

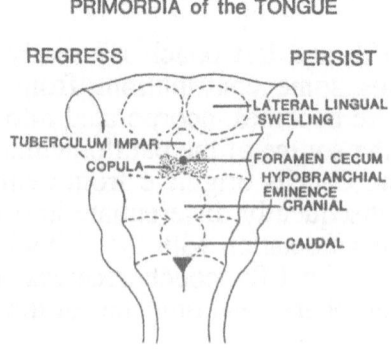

of fusion. The V-shaped line of **circumvallate papillae** near the base of the tongue are stomodeal in origin. The caudal part of the hypobranchial eminence (fourth arch) contributes to the formation of the **epiglottis**. The complex innervation pattern of the adult tongue is explained in the following manner.

1. The mucosa for the anterior two-thirds of the tongue develops from the stomodeal ectoderm of the first branchial arch; this ectodermal area of the oral mucosa receives its general somatic afferent innervation from the trigeminal nerve.

2. Because of the overlapping pattern for general and special afferent innervation in the oropharyngeal mucosa, the first arch area receives its special taste fibers from the facial nerve via the chorda tympani.

3. The mucosa of the posterior one-third of the tongue develops from the pharyngeal endoderm of the third arch (cranial part of hypobranchial eminence); it receives general visceral afferent fibers from the glossopharyngeal and special visceral afferent fibers for taste from the glossopharyngeal nerve and the vagus for the most posterior part of the tongue.

Note: The overlapping innervation pattern is retained by all of the arches but it is obvious only for the first because the chorda tympani can be seen arching over the tympanic membrane. It is not obvious for the other arches because the grooves disappear and the pouches lose their pharyngeal connections.

4. The hypoglossal nerve follows the migrating occipital myoblasts and supplies their general somatic efferent innervation as they differentiate to form all of the intrinsic and extrinsic muscles of the tongue.

QUESTIONS: Chapter 13 - Differentiation of the Branchial Apparatus

1. Which of the following bones does **NOT** originate by endochondral ossification of a branchial arch skeletal element?
   A. mandible
   B. malleus
   C. incus
   D. stapes
   E. hyoid

2. The palatine tonsil is usually considered to develop in association with pharyngeal pouch:
   A. one
   B. two
   C. three
   D. four
   E. five (ultimobranchial body)

3. The thymic lymphocytes originate from:
   A. endoderm of pharyngeal pouch two
   B. ectoderm of branchial groove two
   C. endoderm of pharyngeal pouch three
   D. ectoderm of branchial groove three
   E. none of the above

4. The parenchymal cells of the superior and inferior parathyroid glands originate from the endodermal cells of pharyngeal pouches:
   A. one and two
   B. two and three
   C. three and four
   D. four and five (ultimobranchial body)
   E. none of the above combinations is correct

5. The nerve innervating the branchiomeric musculature derived from the first branchial arch is the:
   A. ophthalmic division of the trigeminal
   B. maxillary division of the trigeminal
   C. mandibular division of the trigeminal
   D. facial
   E. all of the above

6. Cervical cysts are thought to originate from epithelialized remnants of the:
   A. first branchial groove
   B. fourth pharyngeal pouch
   C. thyroglossal duct
   D. cervical sinus
   E. otic vesicle

Answers: 1=A; 2=B; 3=E; 4=C; 5=C; 6=D

CHAPTER 14: FACE AND PALATE

DEVELOPMENT OF THE FACE

Primordia for the upper part of the face are derived primarily from structures developing in association with the forebrain (cerebral hemispheres and eyes); those for the power part of the face (upper and lower jaws) are derived almost entirely from the first branchial arch. Initially, all of the facial primordia surround the stomodeum and form the boundaries of the primitive oral opening; these primordia are the: **frontonasal prominence, maxillary prominences** and the **mandibular prominences.**

Frontonasal Prominence. The superior boundary of the primitive oral opening is formed by the unpaired frontonasal prominence; it will ultimately form facial areas above the external nares and tip of the nose. Most of the structures developing from the frontonasal prominence will be innervated by the **ophthalmic division (V_1)** of the trigeminal nerve.

Maxillary Prominences. The lateral boundaries of the stomodeum are formed by the paired maxillary portions of the first branchial arch; they will ultimately form most of the facial areas between the external nares and superior boundary of the definitive oral opening, i.e., upper jaw. The **maxillary division (V_2)** of the trigeminal nerve will supply almost all of the structures developing from the maxillary portion of the first branchial arch.

Mandibular Prominences. The inferior boundary of the primitive oral cavity is formed by the paired mandibular portions of the first branchial arch; they will ultimately form facial areas below the definitive oral opening. Structures originating from this primordium will be innervated by the **mandibular division (V_3)** of the trigeminal nerve.

Development of suborbital facial areas is intimately associated with the appearance of **nasal (olfactory) placodes** in the inferior (nasal) portion of the frontonasal prominence. These placodes originate as localized thickenings in the superficial ectoderm immediately above the nasolacrimal groove separating the frontonasal and maxillary prominences. A short time later, accumulations of mesenchyme around the periphery of the placodes elevates the adjacent ectoderm above the placode to produce the **nasal pit.** Rapid proliferation of mesenchymal cells in the elevations enclosing the superior aspect of the nasal pit soon produces the prominent **lateral** and **medial nasal prominences.** Although both prominences contribute to formation of the lateral and medial boundaries of the external nares, only the medial prominences will contribute to structures below the tip of the nose, i.e., philtrum and primary palate. The more extensive contributions made to facial development by the medial nasal prominences are reflected by their extension into the central area of the stomodeum.

FACIAL DEVELOPMENT

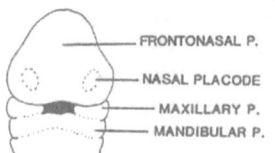

FRONTONASAL P.
NASAL PLACODE
MAXILLARY P.
MANDIBULAR P.

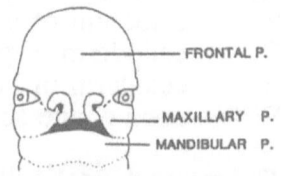

FRONTAL P.
MAXILLARY P.
MANDIBULAR P.

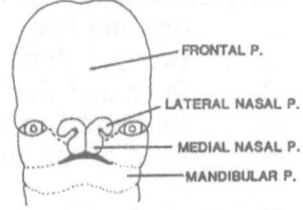

FRONTAL P.
LATERAL NASAL P.
MEDIAL NASAL P.
MANDIBULAR P.

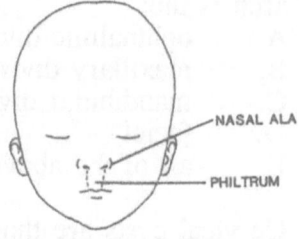

NASAL ALA
PHILTRUM

DIFFERENTIATION OF THE FRONTONASAL PROMINENCES

The superior (frontal) portion of the frontonasal prominence will form the **frontal** (forehead) and **interorbital areas** of the face and the **dorsum of the nose**; near the midline, significant contributions are also made to the supra- and infraorbital areas. The inferior (nasal) portion of the frontonasal prominence contains the nasal placodes with their associated nasal prominences; subsequent differentiation of the lateral and medial nasal prominences and formation of the upper jaw requires contact and fusion with the subjacent maxillary prominences.

Nasal Placodes. Centrally directed processes of bipolar neuroblasts (primary sensory neurons) differentiating in placode epithelium grow into the underlying telencephalon and ultimately make synaptic connections with secondary sensory neurons developing in the olfactory lobes; the distal processes remain exposed on the surface and are very short because the neurons themselves form part of the surface epithelium. Intraepithelial neurons are a primitive condition and explains why the olfactory (I) nerves do not possess sensory ganglia; olfactory neurons retain a bipolar morphology throughout life. After development of the nose is complete, the olfactory epithelium of the nasal placodes will be located in the upper recesses of the nasal cavities.

Lateral Nasal Prominences. As the subjacent maxillary prominences grow toward the midline, mesenchymal infilling obliterates the intervening nasolacrimal groove and brings the maxillary and lateral nasal prominences into apposition; after contact and fusion, the lateral nasal prominences form the sides of the nose, i.e., **nasal alae**.

Medial Nasal Prominences. As facial development progresses, the medial nasal prominences appear to merge or coalesce to form the right and left halves of the very prominent **median nasal prominence**. Continuing growth of the maxillary prominences toward the midline eventually brings them into contact with the centrally located median nasal prominence and when fusion has been effected, the median nasal and maxillary prominences form the central and lateral areas of the upper jaw primordium. Post-fusion stages of median nasal prominence differentiation will be covered with the maxillary prominences because both structures make superficial contributions to the face (upper lip) and deep contributions to the upper jaw and palate. It should be noted that fusion of the maxillary and median nasal prominences also forms the definitive boundaries for the external nares; the definitive lateral (alar) and medial (septal) boundaries are formed, respectively, by the lateral and median nasal prominences; the intervening areas are formed by the maxillary prominences.

DIFFERENTIATION OF THE MEDIAN NASAL AND MAXILLARY PROMINENCES

The primordium for the upper jaw and superior boundary of the definitive oral opening is formed by fusion of the maxillary and median nasal prominences. A short time later, a thickened band of stomodeal ectoderm appears in the jaw primordium and grows into the underlying mesenchyme; this semicircular-shaped band of stomodeal ectoderm is the **labial lamina**. Subsequent degeneration of the central cells of the lamina separates the jaw primordium into **superficial areas** for the face and **deep areas** for the bones of the upper jaw and palate. The space produced within the labial lamina will persist through life as the upper part of the **buccal cavity**; the persisting epithelial cells of the labial lamina will form the mucosal surfaces for the upper lip and adjacent bony structures, i.e., **gingiva**.

Superficial Contributions. The labial or superficial portion of the median nasal prominence forms the **philtrum** or **central area** of the upper lip while **lateral areas** are formed by the superficial part of the maxillary prominences

Deep Contributions. Ultimately, the deep portions of the median nasal prominence will differentiate to form the:

1. **medial portion of the maxilla** (premaxilla) which is associated with incisor teeth, i.e., the intermaxillary portion of the adult human maxilla.

2. **primary palate** (median palatine process) and the nasal septum.

Deep portions of the maxillary prominences will ultimately differentiation to form the:

1. **lateral portion of the maxilla** (maxilla proper) which is associated with the canine and post-canine (premolars and molars) teeth.

2. **secondary palate** (lateral palatine processes).

Note: In vertebrates (except man), the central area of the upper jaw is formed by separate bones called premaxillae and the palatine processes of the premaxillae form the primary or primitive palate. In all mammals with incisors, these teeth develop in association with the premaxillae. Although premaxillae develop within the deep part of the median nasal prominence of human embryos, the sutures between the premaxillae and maxillae disappears before birth. As a consequence of this early fusion, humans do not possess separate premaxillary and maxillary bones; gross anatomists refer to the premaxillary area with the incisor teeth as the intermaxillary portion of the maxilla. This bit of evolutionary history is very important because unilateral and bilateral clefts occurring in this area are the result of fusion failures between the median nasal prominence and the maxillary prominence.

DIFFERENTIATION OF THE MANDIBULAR PROMINENCES

The mandibular portions of the first branchial arch fuse across the midline to form primordium of the lower jaw and inferior boundary of the definitive oral opening. A **labial lamina** comparable to that appearing in the upper jaw separates the mandibular prominences into **superficial** areas for the face (lower lip) and **deep** areas for the mandible and its associated dental structures (teeth and gingiva); labial and dental areas of the mandible are separated by the lower part of the **buccal cavity**.

Note: The labial laminae for the upper and lower jaws develop during the seventh week and their appearance coincides with that of the dental lamina. In some areas of the stomodeum, the labial and dental laminae are in close proximity but both can be identified readily as separate and independent structures; in other areas, however, the epithelial components are in such close proximity that they appear to originate from a common labiodental lamina.

DEVELOPMENT OF THE PALATE

The definitive palate separating the dorsal (respiratory) and ventral (digestive) passages at stomodeal levels is formed by fusion of the primary and secondary palates.

The **primary palate** is a wedge-shaped structure originating from the deep portion of the median nasal prominence, i.e., the palatine process.

The **secondary palate** is formed by fusion of the lateral palatine processes originating from the deep portion of the maxillary prominences.

The initial fusion occurs rostrally between the right and left sides of the median palatine process and the cranial ends of the lateral palatine processes; the fusion then progresses caudally to meet at the apex of the wedge, i.e., future incisive area. Subsequent fusions caudal to the incisive area involves only the lateral palatine prominences and the inferior edge of the nasal septum; the **palatine raphe** permanently marks the fusion site of the lateral palatine process. In the adult, the **incisive papilla** indicates the approximate boundary between the primary and secondary palates; in macerated skulls, the landmark is the **incisive foramen**.

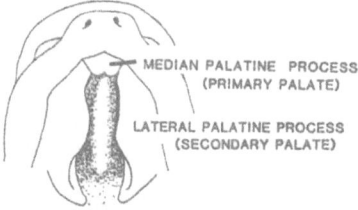

PALATE FORMATION

MEDIAN PALATINE PROCESS (PRIMARY PALATE)

LATERAL PALATINE PROCESS (SECONDARY PALATE)

DEVELOPMENTAL DEFECTS

Developmental defects involving only the superior portion of the frontonasal prominence are relatively rare unless there is an associated open neural tube defect (myeloschisis) of the forebrain. In anencephaly, the frontal bones do not develop but the orbital areas are relatively normal if the eyes are present; absence of frontal bones can be explained by inadequate amount of neural crest mesenchyme and/or an induction failure due to the absence of underlying neural tissue. Oblique facial clefts are produced by persistence of the deep nasolacrimal groove which initially separates the frontonasal and maxillary prominences; in extreme cases, the cleft may reach the upper boundary of the nares and/or the oral opening and the nasolacrimal duct may be incomplete or

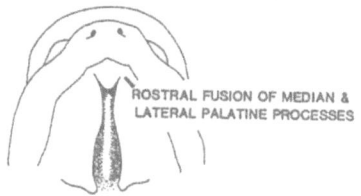

ROSTRAL FUSION OF MEDIAN & LATERAL PALATINE PROCESSES

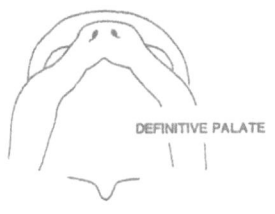

DEFINITIVE PALATE

missing. Labial and palatal clefts are relatively common developmental defects and although either may occur alone, they are frequently present as complete labial-palatal clefts. Almost all unilateral and bilateral clefts are caused by fusion failures between the median nasal and maxillary prominences. If only the superficial or facial (labial) portions of these prominences are involved (incomplete fusion) a simple cleft lip will result; if the deep or palatine components are also involved (complete fusion failure) the result is a cleft lip with a cleft palate. Palatal clefts caudal to the incisive papilla are produced when lateral palatine processes only are involved. Although the olfactory placodes are rather small and insignificant appearing structures, they appear to play a major role in differentiation of the face (nose, upper jaw and palate). Perhaps even more surprising is their suspected role in bilateral differentiation of the telencephalon; paired nasal placodes are thought to be required for differentiation of the right and left cerebral hemispheres, i.e., bilaterality. When the placodes fail to appear or when medial displacement results in formation of a single midline placode, facial and forebrain development are grossly abnormal.

FACIAL MUSCULATURE

It should be noted that the facial areas developing from the frontonasal prominence and first branchial arch (maxillary and mandibular prominences) are secondarily invaded by myoblasts originating from the second arch; however, migration of second arch myoblasts is not limited to the face and other parts of the head. Extensive migrations of facial myoblasts into cervical and upper thoracic levels are known to occur, e.g., platysma. During these migrations, the branchiomeric mesenchyme of the second arch retains its original innervation by the facial (VII) nerve as it differentiates into the muscles of facial expression. The branchiomeric mesenchyme of the mandibular prominence differentiates into the masticatory muscles and retains it innervation from the mandibular division (V_3) of the trigeminal nerve.

FACIAL DEVELOPMENT DURING FETAL LIFE

Complete facial development occurs slowly and is effected primarily by changes in the proportion and relative positions of the five primordia. Enlargement of the developing brain (especially the telencephalon) produces a prominent forehead and appears to be instrumental in moving the laterally placed eyes to their definitive frontal position. Differentiation of the mandibular prominences forming the lower jaw appears to elevate the ears.

QUESTIONS: Chapter 14 - Face and Palate

1. In unilateral clefts of the lip and palate, the course of the cleft passes through the dental (alveolar) arch between:
    A. the right and left medial incisors
    B. the medial and lateral incisors
    C. lateral incisors and canines
    D. canines and post canine teeth

2. Failure of the lateral palatine processes to fuse cross the midline produces:
    A. an oblique facial cleft
    B. an unclosed or defective nasolacrimal duct
    C. a simple midline cleft (true hair lip)
    D. a simple unilateral cleft lip
    E. a simple cleft of the secondary palate

3. A cleft involving the lip and dental arch (alveolar ridge) is produced by fusion failure between the:
    A. mandibular and maxillary prominences
    B. median (medial) nasal and maxillary prominences
    C. lateral nasal and maxillary prominences
    D. right and left maxillary prominences
    E. none of the above

4. When considering the developmental origin of the lateral palatine processes, the definitive palate would be expected to receive all or almost all of its afferent innervation via the:
    A. ophthalmic division of the trigeminal nerve
    B. maxillary division of the trigeminal nerve
    C. mandibular division of the trigeminal nerve
    D. facial nerve
    E. none of the above

5. The sensory innervation of the frontonasal prominence is provided by the:
    A. facial nerve.
    B. ophthalmic division of the trigeminal nerve.
    C. maxillary division of the trigeminal nerve.
    D. mandibular division of the trigeminal nerve.
    E. glossopharyngeal nerve.

6. The median nasal prominence (intermaxillary segment) will form the:
    A. nasal ala
    B. medial portion of the maxilla (premaxilla)
    C. secondary palate
    D. lateral palatine processes
    E. all of the above

Answers: 1=C; 2=E; 3=B; 4=B; 5=B; 6=B

CHAPTER 15: DIGESTIVE SYSTEM AND MESENTERIES

PRIMITIVE GUT

The digestive system is derived almost entirely from the splanchnopleura of the yolk sac roof and acquires its basic tubular configuration as a result of body fold formation (head, tail, lateral); primitive **foregut**, **midgut** and **hindgut** regions are identifiable by the fourth week of development. The endoderm of the primitive gut will persist to form the epithelial **parenchyma** for all segments of the definitive gut, for all parts of the respiratory system caudal to the stomodeum, and for the accessory digestive glands (liver and pancreas); **stromal elements** for all of these structures will differentiate from the associated layer of splanchnic mesoderm. The most cephalic levels of the oral cavity and caudal levels of the anal canal do not originate from the primitive gut; the ectodermal epithelium in these areas is derived from the **stomodeum** and **proctodeum**, respectively.

PRIMITIVE MESENTERIES

Dorsal Mesentery. After coelom formation and development of the body folds, the tubular gut is suspended from the dorsal midline of the body wall by double layers of splanchnic mesoderm which form the **primitive dorsal mesentery.** After gut rotation, the original midline attachment of the primitive dorsal mesentery will be altered by secondary fusions to produce the attachment sites seen in the definitive dorsal mesentery of the adult. The most cephalic level of the foregut (pharynx) is not associated with a coelomic space and does not, therefore, possess a dorsal mesentery. Specific levels of the dorsal mesentery are identified by the region of gut being supported.

Ventral Mesentery. A ventral connection between the tubular gut and anterior body wall is found only at the caudal or venous end of the embryonic heart; this 'primitive ventral mesentery' is the important developmental landmark known as the **septum transversum.**

DIFFERENTIATION OF THE FOREGUT

During differentiation of the branchial apparatus, the area of the fourth branchial arch serves as the site of origin for the respiratory system. The respiratory primordium is first seen as a midline longitudinal groove in the ventral wall of the pharyngeal foregut; this respiratory primordium is referred to as the **laryngotracheal groove.** The caudal portion of the laryngotracheal groove subsequently becomes separated from the pharyngeal lumen to form a tubular diverticulum known as the **lung bud.** Separation is effected by formation of **laryngotracheal folds** which fuse across the midline to form the **tracheoesophageal septum.** A short time later, partitioning within the septum separates the dorsally located esophagus from the ventral lung bud; the lung bud will ultimately form the trachea, bronchi and lungs. Later stages of respiratory development will be covered in a later chapter.

Note: The terms used to indicate primitive gut areas are convenient descriptive terms only and are used during early development because other anatomical landmarks have not yet developed. During differentiation of the digestive system and in the adult, arterial blood supply is used as the basis for determining definitive foregut, midgut and hindgut levels of the digestive system. The most important arteries used in making these distinctions are the **celiac** (foregut), **superior mesenteric** (midgut) and **inferior mesenteric** (hindgut); some overlap in vasculature does occur in junctional areas of the definitive foregut, midgut and hindgut.

Foregut Derivatives. In craniocaudal sequence, the digestive portion of the foregut forms the posterior one-third of the oral cavity, oropharynx, esophagus, stomach and upper half of the duodenum including the common bile duct and liver as well as the pancreatic ducts and pancreas (endocrine and exocrine).

Vasculature.   Definitive foregut areas are supplied by branches from the external carotids, small vessels arising directly from the thoracic aorta and the celiac artery.

Developmental Defects.   Due to the common origin from the ventral wall of the foregut, defective partitioning by the laryngotracheal folds and/or the tracheoesophageal septum may give rise to stenotic and/or atretic segments in one or both structures or to fistulous connections between the trachea and esophagus.

DIFFERENTIATION OF THE MIDGUT

The definitive arrangement of abdominal viscera and mesenteries is the result of gut rotation followed by changes in attachment sites for the primitive dorsal mesentery; the latter process is referred to as **gut fixation**. During fixation, the mesentery of the gut segment being "fixed" is lost by fusion with the peritoneum covering adjacent areas of the body wall and in the process, the corresponding gut segment usually becomes **retroperitoneal**.

Gut Rotation.   When viewed from the ventral aspect, the adult configuration of the abdominal viscera is produced by a single, counterclockwise rotation of approximately 270 degrees. The segment of gut undergoing rotation is referred to as the **midgut loop**. The **axis** for rotation of the midgut loop is formed by the superior mesenteric and stalk of the yolk sac; the axial structures are used to delineate **cranial** and **caudal** limbs of the midgut loop. Complete rotation occurs over a period of several weeks and occurs in two phases; the most significant events occurring in the two phases are:

1.   **physiological herniation** of the midgut loop into the umbilical coelom.

2.   **return (retraction)** of the midgut loop into the embryonic abdominal cavity.

Herniation Phase.   Although herniation of the midgut loop into the umbilical coelom may be facilitated by attachment of the yolk stalk to the umbilical cord, herniation is usually attributed to difficulties arising from the need to accommodate a rapidly growing gut in a slowly enlarging abdominal cavity and as a consequence of the size discrepancy, the midgut loop grows into the adjacent spaced provided by the umbilical portion of the extraembryonic coelom. Within the umbilical coelom, the midgut loop undergoes an initial rotation of 90

GUT ROTATION & DEVELOPMENT

HERNIATED MIDGUT LOOP

S. MESENTERIC
CRANIAL LIMB
HINDGUT
YOLK STALK   CAUDAL LIMB

RETURN BEGINNING

DUODENUM
CAUDAL LIMB
HINDGUT
YOLK STALK   CRANIAL LIMB

RETURN COMPLETE

CECUM
INTESTINAL COILS
TERMINAL ILEUM   HINDGUT

GUT ROTATION COMPLETE

SPLENIC FLEXURE
HEPATIC FLEXURE
HINDGUT
ASCENDING COLON

degrees, i.e., cranial limb to the right, caudal limb to the left. Following the initial rotation, temporary intestinal coils begin to form in the cranial limb; the cecal diverticulum appears in the caudal limb a short time later.

Return Phase. Degeneration of the yolk stalk normally occurs at this time, but its persistence does not prevent retraction. The cranial limb begins to retract first and resumes its counterclockwise rotation of 180 degrees to pass down and under the rotational axis (superior mesenteric) and under the more slowly developing caudal limb.

Retraction appears to be accomplished by the formation of a second group of intra-abdominal intestinal coils located in the region of the future duodenojejunal junction. As the number of intra-abdominal coils increase, there is a corresponding decrease in the number of umbilical coils until all of the cranial limb has been retracted under the superior mesenteric artery and under the more slowly developing caudal limb. The return phase is completed when the lagging caudal limb has returned to the abdominal cavity but gut rotation in not complete until all of the visceral structures have reached their definitive positions. It should be noted that after completion of the return phase, the cecum is still located near the liver in the upper right quadrant. Continuing growth of adjacent areas during the post-return period allows the cecum to descend and eventually reach its definitive location. Gut rotation is complete only when the cecum is positioned in the lower right quadrant of the abdominal cavity.

Midgut Derivatives. The definitive midgut forms the duodenum below the origin of the common bile duct, the jejunum, ileum, cecum, appendix, ascending colon and transverse colon to a point near the splenic flexure; all derivatives begin their differentiation during gut rotation.

Vasculature. Definitive midgut areas are supplied by the superior mesentery artery; some overlap with foregut vasculature (celiac) and hindgut (inferior mesenteric) occurs in junctional areas. **Note:** Despite it dual blood supply, the pancreas is considered to be a foregut derivative; the duodenum however, is considered to be a foregut and a midgut derivative.

Developmental Defects. The presence of abdominal viscera in a persistent umbilical coelom produces an omphalocele and may be the result of incomplete return of the midgut loop. Malrotation and abnormalities in post-rotation fixation may result from incomplete or clockwise rotation; complications which may result from clockwise rotation and/or malrotations with abnormal fixation include: duodenal obstruction, volvulus and intussusception. Remnants of the yolk stalk (Meckel's diverticulum) are found in about 2 percent of the adult population and are usually asymptomatic; they are always located on the antimesenteric border of the ileum about 18-25 inches above the ileocecal junction. Persistence of the entire yolk stalk produces a connection between the terminal ileum and anterior body wall at the umbilicus; the connection may be fibrous, fibrocystic or fistulous if completely canalized. Because the gut lumen is normally occluded during early stages of development, stenosis, atresia and luminal duplications can occur if recanalization fails-to occur or if the recanalization process in abnormal. Although recanalization defects can occur at any level of the gut, they seem to occur most frequently in areas with small luminal diameters during development, e.g., stenosis and/or atresia are more common in the esophagus and small intestine than in the stomach and colon. In newborn infants, stenotic and atretic defects in lower foregut areas (pyloric and duodenal) are frequently associated with projectile vomiting; a clue to the exact level of obstruction may be provided by the presence or absence of bile stained vomitus. Pyloric stenosis can also be the result of pyloric sphincter hypertrophy but this stenotic condition is thought to have a genetic basis and is more prevalent in males. Since high gastrointestinal obstruction also interferes with intestinal reabsorption of amniotic fluid, such obstructions may be associated with polyhydramnios.

DIFFERENTIATION OF THE HINDGUT

During the earliest stages of development, the terminal position of the primitive hindgut is expanded to form the **cloaca**; at this time, the cloaca also forms the terminal portion of the urinary and reproductive systems, i.e., the cloaca forms the terminal portion of the digestive, urinary and reproductive passages. In addition to the communications with these organ systems, the ventral part of the cloaca is in direct communication cranially with the urachal (intra-embryonic) portion of the allantois. Development of the **urorectal septum** or fold and its subsequent fusion with the cloacal membrane divides the common cloacal chamber into dorsal (rectal) and ventral (urogenital) cavities; the same fusion also divides the cloacal membrane into dorsal (anal) and ventral (urogenital) membranes. A short time later, mesodermal cells will accumulate around the periphery of the anal membrane to produce the ectodermally lined anal pit or **proctodeum**; subsequent degeneration of the membrane produces the definitive anal opening and the lower one-third of the anal canal.

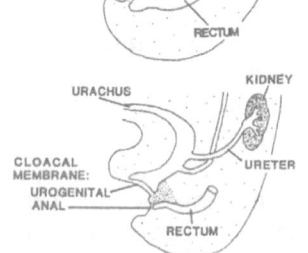

PARTITIONING OF THE HINDGUT

Hindgut Derivatives. The digestive portion of the hindgut contributes to the formation of the descending colon, sigmoid colon, rectum and upper two-thirds of the anal canal; the lower one-third develops from the proctodeum. The junction of endodermal and ectodermal areas is indicated by the **pectinate-line** at the level of the **anal valves**.

Vasculature. Digestive derivatives of the hindgut are supplied by the inferior mesenteric artery with additional contributions to the lower rectum from the middle (internal iliac) and inferior (internal pudendal) hemorrhoidal arteries; some overlap with vasculature of the midgut (superior mesenteric) occurs near the splenic flexure.

Developmental Defects. Abnormalities in formation and fusion of the urorectal septum may result in fistulous connections between the rectum and urogenital sinus with or without abnormal terminations of the urinary and genital ducts. Failure of the anal membrane to rupture results in imperforate anus. Congenital megacolon (Hirschsprung's disease) is caused by defective development of the myenteric plexus and is attributed to failure of migratory neural crest cells to invade the developing musculature. Absence of peristaltic movement in the involved segments creates an obstruction resulting in the accumulation of gut contents in normal gut above the lesion.

ACCESSORY DIGESTIVE STRUCTURES

Pancreas. The pancreas develops from dorsal and ventral evaginations originating from the foregut endoderm. The larger and more cephalic **dorsal bud** grows cranially and extends into the developing greater omentum which now contains the developing **spleen**: this is why the tail of the adult pancreas is usually located in the hilum of the spleen. The smaller and more caudally located ventral outgrowth turns dorsally to reach the duodenal mesentery and fuses with the dorsal outgrowth. After fusion, the duct of the ventral outgrowth becomes the terminal portion of the main pancreatic duct (Wirsung) while that of the dorsal outgrowth persists as the accessory pancreatic duct (Santorini).

The dorsal pancreatic primordium forms almost all of the adult pancreas (upper half of the head, neck, body, tail); the ventral pancreatic primordium forms only the lower part of the head and the uncinate process. The endocrine portion of the pancreas (islets of Langerhans) proliferates as solid epithelial cords from the duct system of the exocrine pancreas; insulin secretion is thought to begin about the middle of gestation.

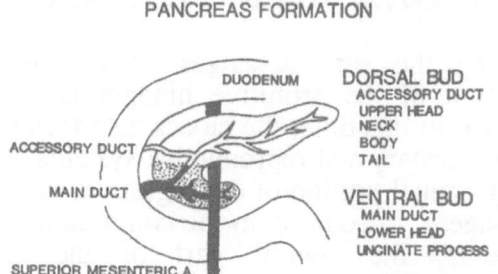

PANCREAS FORMATION

DUODENUM

ACCESSORY DUCT

MAIN DUCT

SUPERIOR MESENTERIC A.

DORSAL BUD
ACCESSORY DUCT
UPPER HEAD
NECK
BODY
TAIL

VENTRAL BUD
MAIN DUCT
LOWER HEAD
UNCINATE PROCESS

The pancreas receives its arterial blood supply via branches from the celiac and superior mesenteric. Despite its dual blood supply from foregut and midgut arteries, it is customary to consider the entire pancreas as a foregut derivative; the duodenum however, is considered to originate from foregut and midgut.

Liver, Gall Bladder and Biliary Ducts. The liver arises as a ventral evagination (**hepatic diverticulum**) from the most caudal level of the foregut epithelium. The diverticulum, which persists throughout life as the **common bile duct**, grows ventrally to invade the mesenchyme of the septum transversum. Vigorous proliferation produces multiple anastomotic cords of developing liver cells (**hepatocytes**) which quickly occupy almost all of the mesenchyme in the caudal portion of the septum transversum (the diaphragm is developing from the cranial portion). As proliferation continues, the rapidly expanding liver and its connecting common bile duct grow beyond the boundaries of the septum carrying with them peritoneal reflections derived from the surface of the septum transversum. The peritoneal fold produced by the common bile duct persists in the adult as the **lesser omentum** with the common bile duct located in its free edge. The septal peritoneum is reflected onto the expanding mass of hepatocytes and persists as the visceral peritoneum of the adult liver and as the ligaments enclosing the bare area of the liver, i.e., **coronary** and **triangular (right and left) ligaments**.

As liver development continues outside the septum transversum, the left umbilical vein is surrounded and slowly pulled away from the anterior body wall carrying with it a peritoneal reflection which persists throughout life as the **falciform ligament**. In the adult, the free edge of the falciform ligament contains a fibrous remnant of the umbilical vein (**ligamentum teres hepatis**) which can be traced from the porta hepatis through the substance of the liver as the **ligamentum venosus**, i.e., the intrahepatic portion of the umbilical vein or ductus venosus .

Hematopoiesis begins in the liver during the second month of development and although the developing **bone marrow** (primary ossification centers) begins to produce blood cells during the third month, hematopoietic foci are still present in the liver at birth. At the beginning of the fetal period (nine weeks), the liver comprises 10 percent of the fetal mass.

The liver receives its arterial blood supply from the hepatic branch of the celiac but the arterial supply is supplemented by blood received via the hepatic portal vein; both arterial and venous blood supplies are required to maintain hepatic viability.

Developmental Defects. Biliary atresia is the most common defect associated with liver development and is caused by failure of the intrahepatic bile ducts to canalize. Comparable canalization defects may occur in pancreas and contribute to the formation of pancreatic cysts.

Salivary Glands. The salivary glands arise as epithelial proliferations from the oral cavity during the sixth and seventh weeks of development. The **parotid** is the first to appear followed by the **submandibular** (submaxillary) and **sublingual** gland complex. The parotid is considered to develop from the stomodeal portion of the oral cavity but, for reasons which are not clear, the submandibular and sublingual gland complex (major and minor glands) are almost invariably listed as originating from foregut endoderm. This interpretation is unusual because the termination of their ducts, which usually indicates the site of origin, and the location of both glands is rostral to the parotid.

FATE OF THE PRIMITIVE DORSAL MESENTERY

Initially, the primitive dorsal mesentery is continuous and suspends the entire length of the primitive gut from the dorsal midline of the body cavity. During gut fixation, however, the continuity is interrupted at several levels and the midline attachment is altered by fusions of the mesentery to peritoneal areas located to the right or left of the median plane. The newly formed mesenteric attachments are frequently referred to as **peritoneal ligaments** and are usually named by the structures connected.

FOREGUT MESENTERIES

Mesoesophagus. Cranial to the septum transversum (future diaphragm), the dorsal mesentery of the foregut is broad and indistinct and at this time, the esophagus with its robust layer of splanchnic mesoderm (including the mesoesophagus) is commonly referred to as the **primitive mediastinum.** The term primitive mediastinum is used to indicate the importance of this area during subsequent partitioning of the coelomic space into separate pericardial, pleural and peritoneal cavities. The splanchnic mesoderm of the mesoesophagus is eventually incorporated into the connective tissues of definitive mediastinal structures.

Mesogastrium (Greater Omentum). The spleen (lien) develops as a localized accumulation of mesenchymal cells around blood vessels located in the mesogastrium; after the spleen appears, the following subdivisions (peritoneal ligaments) can be recognized in the greater omentum.

1. **gastrophrenic** - between the stomach and diaphragm above the spleen
2. **gastrolienal** - between the stomach and spleen
3. **lienorenal** - between the spleen and kidney (sometimes called lienophrenic)
4. **phrenicocolic** (sustentaculum lieni) - between the diaphragm and transverse colon
5. **gastrocolic** - between stomach and transverse colon
6. **omental apron** - covers but is unattached to the remaining abdominal viscera

Mesoduodenum. The dorsal mesentery is lost during fixation when the duodenum and its associated pancreatic primordia become retroperitoneal.

MIDGUT MESENTERIES

Mesentery of the Small Intestine. The definitive mesentery for the jejunum and ileum is derived almost entirely from the mesentery supporting the cranial limb of the midgut loop during gut rotation; a small segment for the terminal ileum originates from the mesentery of the caudal limb.

Mesoappendix. The mesentery of the appendix represents a small and insignificant derivative of the mesentery for the caudal limb of the midgut loop.

Ascending Mesocolon. The mesentery of the ascending colon is normally lost by fixation to the right posterior body wall.

Transverse Mesocolon.   The primitive transverse mesocolon fuses with the posterior fold or leaf of the greater omentum to form the definitive transverse mesocolon of the adult.

HINDGUT MESENTERIES

Descending Mesocolon.   The cephalic portion of the mesentery is normally lost by fixation to the left posterior body wall; caudally, the fusion is not complete.

Sigmoid Mesocolon.   Incomplete fusion allows the caudalmost portion of the descending mesocolon to persist as the mesentery of the sigmoid colon.

FATE OF THE PRIMITIVE VENTRAL MESENTERY (SEPTUM TRANSVERSUM)

Lesser Omentum.   The lesser omentum is a peritoneal reflection formed as the liver and common bile duct grow beyond the confines of the septum transversum; it is comprised of two peritoneal ligaments.

1.   **hepatogastric ligament** - between the liver and lesser curvature of the stomach
2.   **hepatoduodenal ligament** - free edge of the lesser omentum containing the common bile duct, hepatic artery, and portal vein

Hepatic Ligaments.   The hepatic ligaments are peritoneal reflections formed when the liver grows beyond the septum transversum and in the process, separates the umbilical vein from the anterior body wall.

1.   **falciform ligament** - between the anterior body wall and liver; in the adult, its free edge contains the fibrous remnant of the umbilical vein, i.e., ligamentum teres hepatis.

2.   **coronary ligament** - surrounds the bare areas of the liver and diaphragm; the right and left triangular ligaments are part of the coronary ligament.

QUESTIONS: Chapter 15 - Digestive System and Mesenteries

1. The principal axis for gut rotation is the:
   A. body or connecting stalk
   B. septum transversum
   C. caudal limb of the midgut loop
   D. celiac artery
   E. superior mesenteric artery

2. Gut rotation is considered to be complete when:
   A. the yolk stalk disappears
   B. the umbilical coils appear
   C. the cecal diverticulum appears
   D. return of the caudal limb is complete
   E. the cecum is located in the lower right quadrant

3. The landmark used to delineate foregut and midgut contributions to the duodenum is the:
   A. accessory pancreatic duct
   B. main pancreatic duct
   C. common bile duct
   D. duodenal flexure
   E. none of the above

4. The hepatocytes (liver cells) are usually considered to be derived from:
   A. foregut endoderm
   B. mesenchyme of the septum transversum
   C. midgut endoderm
   D. midgut splanchnic mesoderm
   E. mesogastrium

5. Choose the **INCORRECT** statement concerning Meckel's diverticulum.
   A. It is a relatively common gut anomaly.
   B. It is usually attached to the terminal ileum.
   C. It is located within the dorsal mesentery.
   D. It represents a persistent portion of the yolk stalk.
   E. It is sometimes attached to the umbilicus by a fibrous cord.

6. Hirschsprung's disease (congenital megacolon) appears to result from:
   A. clockwise rotation and improper fixation of the midgut loop
   B. almost total absence of smooth muscle in the wall of the colon
   C. failure of the lumen to recanalize, i.e., atresia
   D. failure of neural crest cells to form the myenteric plexus in the affected region of the hindgut
   E. persistence of the cloacal membrane (anal portion only)

Answers: 1=E; 2=E; 3=C; 4=A; 5=C; 6=D

CHAPTER 16: DIAPHRAGM AND BODY CAVITIES

COELOM FORMATION

Coelom formation begins in the trilaminar embryo during the third week of development and coincides with late stages of embryonic mesoderm formation. At this time, the midline axis of the embryo (oral membrane, notochord, cloacal membrane) is devoid of mesoderm and as a consequence, the developing coelom cannot cross the midline in these areas. Coelomic spaces can, however, cross the midline in areas cranial to the oropharyngeal membrane because the embryonic mesoderm will fuse to form the cardiogenic area. Coelom formation is essentially complete by the beginning of the fourth week and its basic **shape, boundaries** and **communications** with the extraembryonic coelom are established before the first somite appears (about 21 days).

Coelomic Shape. The first evidence of impending coelom formation appears laterally and is indicated by the appearance of small isolated spaces within the growing sheets of embryonic mesoderm. Expansion and coalescence of the isolated spaces soon produce larger but noncommunicating right and left coelomic cavities; continuity between the lateral spaces is established by progressive extension and incorporation of midline coelomic spaces appearing in the cardiogenic mesoderm. Coelomic continuity across the midline produces a single body cavity and produces the basic inverted "U" configuration of the completely formed embryonic coelom.

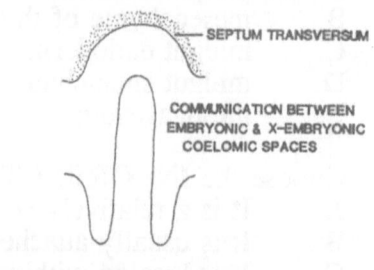

BODY CAVITY FORMATION

DORSAL VIEW BEFORE FOLDING

Coelomic Boundaries. Development of the coelomic space divides the embryonic mesoderm into somatic and splanchnic layers which will form the boundaries for all parts of the coelomic cavity (pericardial, pleural, peritoneal) throughout life. Subsequently, the somatic and splanchnic layers become permanently associated with the adjacent layers of ectoderm and endoderm to form, respectively, the somatopleura of the primitive body wall and the splanchnopleura of the primitive gut wall. It should be noted, that it is actually the appearance of a coelom that first delineates areas of lateral plate and paraxial mesoderm in the embryo.

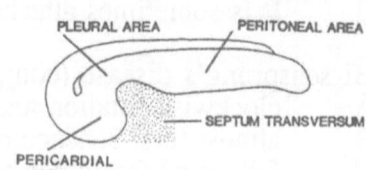

LATERAL VIEW AFTER FOLDING

Coelomic Communications. After the shape and boundaries of the embryonic coelom have been formed the lateral arms of the coelom continue to expand peripherally and upon reaching the edge of the embryonic plate, they establish broad bilateral communications with the previously formed extraembryonic coelom. These areas of communication between the embryonic and extraembryonic spaces are important because they will ultimately be located at the umbilicus and allow the herniating midgut loop access to the adjacent umbilical coelom.

It must be emphasized that a comparable peripheral expansion of the coelom does not occur in the midline cardiogenic area and that as a consequence, the pericardial and extraembryonic cavities remain separated by a band of embryonic mesoderm called the **septum transversum**. At this time, the septum transversum is the most cephalic structure of the embryonic disk and forms the superior boundary of the pericardial cavity; these relationships will be reversed after head fold formation.

Significance of the Septum Transversum. The septum transversum is one of the earliest permanent landmarks to form during development and it is particularly important because from the time of its appearance, the septum transversum will always define either the cranial (before head fold formation) or caudal (after head fold formation) boundary of the pericardial cavity. Furthermore, since the mesoderm forming the septum is not split into somatic and splanchnic layers by coelom formation, it persists as a permanent connection between the body (somatopleura) and gut (splanchnopleura) walls; it is this persistent connection that allows the septum to function as a very broad but short 'ventral mesentery'. Because of its strategic location with respect to the heart, gut and coelomic spaces, some of its important features and contributions are summarized below.

1. The septal mesoderm forms a major portion of the definitive diaphragm separating the peritoneal from the pleural and pericardial cavities; lesser but important contributions are made to the membranes effecting separation of the definitive pericardial and pleural cavities. The skeletal muscle of the diaphragm is, however, derived from cervical myotomes.

2. Caudally, the septal mesoderm forms all of the connective tissue stroma for the liver (Glisson's capsule) and for the hepatic associated peritoneal ligaments, e.g., lesser omentum and coronary ligaments.

3. During the early stages of cardiovascular development, all veins returning blood to the heart must traverse the septum transversum to reach the sinus venosus.

When coelom formation is complete, the entire coelomic space of the trilaminar embryo lies in a single plane, has the configuration of an inverted "U" and its cranial boundary is formed by the septum transversum. During head fold formation, which involves all parts of the embryo cranial to the notochord, the bend of the "U" is folded ventrally and caudally to bring the pericardial cavity into its definitive position anterior to the foregut and with the septum transversum now forming its caudal or diaphragmatic boundary. The two arms of the "U" are not involved in the folding process and retain a dorsal position with the gut. The portions of the embryonic coelom dorsal to the septum transversum will form the pleural and peritoneal cavities. During subsequent stages of partitioning, the:

1. **pericardial cavity** will develop from the folded or ventral part of the coelomic space.

2. **pleural cavities** will develop from the dorsal portion of the coelomic space cranial to the septum transversum, i.e., immediately dorsal to the pericardial cavity.

3. **peritoneal cavity** will develop from the dorsal portion of the coelomic space caudal to the septum transversum.

PARTITIONING OF THE COELOMIC SPACE

PERICARDIAL CAVITY

Separation of the pericardial cavity from the dorsally located pleural/peritoneal space is effected by the formation of right and left **pleuropericardial membranes** or folds. Development of pleuropericardial membranes appears to be closely associated with cardiovascular development because the common cardinal veins (ducts of Cuvier) are located in the free edges of the developing membranes. The folds originate from the lateral body wall and adjacent areas of the septum transversum and grow medially to fuse with the splanchnic mesoderm of the ventral wall of the esophagus, i.e., a **ventral fusion** with the primitive mediastinum.

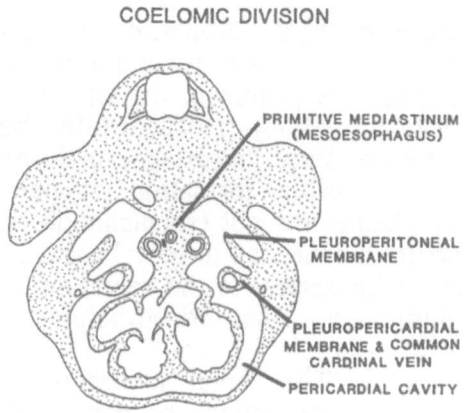

COELOMIC DIVISION

PRIMITIVE MEDIASTINUM (MESOESOPHAGUS)

PLEUROPERITONEAL MEMBRANE

PLEUROPERICARDIAL MEMBRANE & COMMON CARDINAL VEIN

PERICARDIAL CAVITY

Developmental Defects. Abnormalities associated with pleuropericardial membrane development are rare and the rarity is attributed to their relationship with the developmentally important common cardinal veins. Communications between the pericardial and pleural cavities in the adult are almost invariably acquired secondarily as the result of some disease process.

Note: Most of the 'definitive pleuropericardial membranes' separating the heart and lungs of the adult (mediastinal pleura and parietal pericardium) are new structures split from the internal surface of the body wall by the developing lungs; the embryonic or original pleuropericardial membranes form only the dorsal attachment sites for the membranous structures of the adult. It is the lateral and ventral expansion of the lungs and pleural cavities within the body wall that moves the heart and pericardial cavity to its definitive location in the mediastinum and allows the pleural structures to eventually become the most anterior visceral structures in the thorax. The splitting process within the body wall is also responsible for moving the **phrenic nerve** from its original somatopleuric location to its definitive position between the parietal pericardium and the mediastinal pleura.

PLEURAL AND PERITONEAL CAVITIES

Separation of the pleural and peritoneal cavities is effected by the formation of right and left **pleuroperitoneal membranes**. These membranes originate from the lateral body wall and dorsal edge of the septum transversum and grow dorsomedially to fuse with the splanchnic mesoderm of the dorsal wall of the esophagus (mesoesophagus), i.e., a **dorsal fusion** with the primitive mediastinum.

Developmental Defects. Formation of the pleuroperitoneal membranes appears to be an independent growth process not associated with the development of other structures and as a consequence, developmental defects are relatively common. Defects involving the pleuroperitoneal membranes are always dorsal and are almost invariably found on the left side (comparable defects on the right are less vulnerable to herniation of abdominal viscera because of the protection provided by greater development of the right side of the liver). The defects range from slight muscular defects producing a thin membranous costovertebral trigone in the diaphragm to persistence of a common pleuro/peritoneal cavity. Herniation of abdominal viscera (with or without membranous sacs) may compromise fetal lung development and result in moderate to severe pulmonary hypoplasia.

DIAPHRAGM FORMATION

The definitive diaphragm of the adult receives contributions from the following structures:

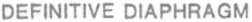

1. septum transversum
2. pleuroperitoneal membranes
3. splanchnic mesoderm surrounding the esophagus (primitive mediastinum)
4. body wall (produced as a result of lung and pleural cavity growth within the somatopleura); these areas receive their sensory innervation via somatopleuric intercostal nerves.

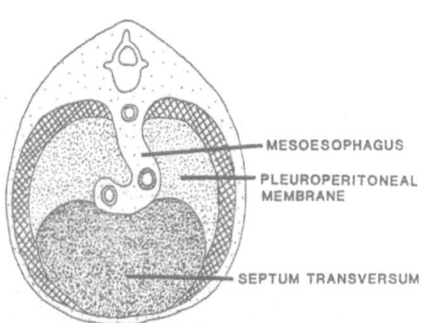

Note: The skeletal muscle for all parts of the diaphragm is derived from cervical myotomes (primarily C-4); the septum transversum allows migrating myoblasts in the somatopleura to extend across the coelomic space, reach the wall of the foregut and ultimately differentiate into the crura of the diaphragm surrounding the esophageal hiatus.

QUESTIONS: Chapter 16 - Diaphragm and Body Cavities

1. Developmental defects of the diaphragm are usually:
    A. bilateral and dorsal
    B. bilateral and ventral
    C. unilateral (left) and ventral
    D. unilateral (left) and dorsal
    E. unilateral (right) and dorsal

2. A clue to the earliest position of the developing diaphragm is provided by its:
    A. relationship to the common cardinal veins (ducts of Cuvier)
    B. perforation by the esophagus, thoracic aorta and inferior vena cava
    C. close proximity to the liver
    D. innervation by spinal nerves originating from cervical levels
    E. all of the above

3. Developmental defects involving the pleuropericardial membrane are rare but, when they occur, the developmental basis is a failure of the pleuropericardial membrane to fuse with the:
    A. ventral part of the esophageal mesoderm
    B. pleuropericardial membrane of the opposite side
    C. septum transversum
    D. dorsal mesentery of the esophagus
    E. somatopleura

4. Congenital diaphragmatic hernia involving a posterolateral defect in the diaphragm usually results from a failure of the left pleuroperitoneal membrane to fuse with the:
    A. pleuroperitoneal membrane on the right
    B. dorsal mesentery of the esophagus
    C. fibrous pericardium
    D. somatopleura
    E. cervical myotomes on the right

5. After formation of the head fold, the:
    A. pericardial cavity is located ventral to the foregut
    B. pericardial cavity is limited caudally by the septum transversum
    C. heart is suspended from the floor of the foregut by the mesocardium
    D. original polarity of the heart tube has been reversed
    E. all of the above

6. The definitive diaphragm does **NOT** receive contributions from the:
    A. pleuropericardial membranes
    B. pleuroperitoneal membranes
    C. septum transversum
    D. body wall
    E. primitive mediastinum (esophagus and mesoesophagus)

Answers: 1=D; 2=D; 3=A; 4=B; 5=E; 6=A

CHAPTER 17: RESPIRATORY SYSTEM

Development of the upper portion of the respiratory system is closely associated with formation of the face (external nares), stomodeum (nasal cavities) and cephalic levels of the pharyngeal foregut (nasopharynx); the lower respiratory passages (larynx, trachea, bronchi) and lungs develop from a respiratory primordium originating from the ventral wall of the pharynx.

UPPER RESPIRATORY PASSAGES

The lateral and medial boundaries of the future external nares are established during facial development by the appearance of **nasal placodes** in the inferior portion of the **frontonasal prominence** and subsequent formation of the **lateral and medial nasal prominences**; the definitive boundaries are completed by fusion of the maxillary and median nasal prominences during formation of the upper jaw. The paired, ectodermally lined **nasal cavities** originate from the stomodeum. Partitioning of the stomodeum into respiratory (dorsal) and digestive (ventral) passages is effected by development and fusion of lateral palatine processes ; like the median palatine prominence, the septum separating the paired nasal cavities develops from the deep portion of the median nasal prominence and is formed during palate formation. The approximate dividing line between ectoderm (stomodeum) and endodermal (foregut) contributions to the upper respiratory passages is near the caudal edge of the hard palate; in purely respiratory areas, both differentiate to form **ciliated, pseudostratified columnar epithelium**, i.e., classical respiratory epithelium.

NASAL PLACODE

After development of the face and partitioning of the stomodeum are well advanced, the neuroectoderm of the nasal placodes is located in the upper recesses of the paired nasal cavities. Some of the placode epithelial cells differentiate into bipolar olfactory neurons which contribute processes to form the multiple rootlets of the olfactory nerves; subsequent formation of bone around the rootlets is responsible for the many small foramina seen in the cribiform plate of the adult ethmoid bone. The remaining placode cells differentiate to form the basal and sustentacular cells of the olfactory epithelium.

LOWER RESPIRATORY PASSAGES

The primordium for the lower portion of the respiratory system appears during differentiation of the branchial apparatus and is first seen as a midline **laryngotracheal groove** in the floor of the pharyngeal foregut. The upper end of the laryngotracheal groove is located in the area of the fourth branchial arch caudal to the hypobranchial eminence. At its origin, the groove remains in open communication with the pharynx but the caudal portion of the groove becomes separated to form a ventral respiratory primordium known as the **lung bud**. Separation of the respiratory primordium from the pharyngeal foregut is effected by the formation of **laryngotracheal folds** which subsequently fuse across the midline to form a **tracheoesophageal septum**. A short time later, intraseptal splitting separates the dorsally located esophagus from the ventral respiratory primordium; the respiratory primordium will ultimately form the **larynx, trachea, bronchi** and **lungs**.

LOWER AIRWAY DEVELOPMENT

LARYNGOTRACHEAL FOLD & GROOVE

LUNG BUDS (PRIMARY BRONCHI)

ESOPHAGUS

TRACHEA

RIGHT LOBAR BRONCHI

LEFT LOBAR BRONCHI

LARYNX

The communication between the laryngotracheal groove and pharyngeal lumen persists as the laryngeal orifice or **glottis**; the **epiglottis** is formed by the adjacent hypobranchial eminence (caudal part). Skeletal elements of branchial arches four, five and six are thought to form the laryngeal cartilages (thyroid, arytenoid, cricoid); the laryngeal musculature appears to originate from branchial arches four and six only. The **cricothyroid** muscle is innervated by the superior laryngeal branch of the vagus and is apparently the only laryngeal muscle derived from arch four; all of the other laryngeal muscles are innervated by the accessory nerve via its contributions to the inferior (recurrent) laryngeal branch of the vagus. It should be noted that the branchiomeric mesenchyme of the caudal arches also contributes skeletal muscle to the pharynx (constrictors), upper half of the esophagus; the sixth also makes large contributions to the pectoral girdle (trapezius and sternocleidomastoid).

TRACHEA, BRONCHI AND LUNGS

The caudal end of the laryngotracheal groove which was converted into a tubular structure by formation of the tracheoesophageal septum represents the primordium of the trachea, bronchi and lungs. The tubular diverticulum grows caudally and bifurcates to produce the right and left lung buds which will ultimately form the **primary bronchi** for the definitive lung. As lateral growth of the bronchial divisions continues, they project into the pleural portion of the embryonic coelom and carry with them a layer of splanchnic mesoderm which forms the **visceral pleura** and other stromal elements for the lung. Subsequently, the right and left lung branch again to produce the **secondary bronchi** for the lobes of the lungs (three on the right, two on the left). Repeated divisions of the secondary or lobar bronchi produce the **tertiary** or **segmental bronchi**; distal growth with branching produces additional generations of bronchi, bronchioles, terminal bronchioles, respiratory bronchioles and finally the terminal sacs of the 'primitive alveoli'. Alveolar ducts and mature alveoli of the adult lung develop after birth.

DIFFERENTIATION OF THE LUNG

Lung development is usually divided into four stages which may overlap by several weeks because differentiation in the apical portions of the lung occurs earlier than comparable changes in the basal areas.

STAGE 1: **Glandular or Pseudoglandular Period** (weeks 5-17)
Only the conducting system develops during this stage, i.e., through the terminal bronchioles.

STAGE 2: **Canalicular Period** (weeks 13-25)
Luminal diameter of the conducting system increases and development of respiratory areas (respiratory bronchioles) begins. At the end of this period, a few terminal sacs with flattened epithelium (primitive alveoli) begin to appear.

STAGE 3: **Terminal Sac Period** (weeks 24 to birth)
As the name implies, this period is characterized by the development of large numbers of terminal sacs and is accompanied by a marked increase in vascularity.

By the 28th week of development, the respiratory area and vascularity are adequate for survival of premature infants. Surface area for gaseous exchange and vascularity appear to be more important to survival than epithelial flattening, i.e., differentiation of **alveolar type I** epithelial cells. Surfactant producing **alveolar type II** cells begin to appear at about 28 weeks. **Note:** Terminal sacs or 'primitive alveoli' are considered to correspond to the alveolar ducts of the adult lung.

STAGE 4:   **Alveolar Period** (late fetal to 8 years)
During infancy and early childhood, the number of primitive alveoli is increased by distal proliferation as the more proximal areas differentiate into alveolar ducts and mature alveoli. The rate of proliferation declines during late childhood when the rate of maturation begins to exceed the rate of proliferation. Unlike primitive alveoli, the mature alveoli cannot proliferate to form new generations of alveoli.

Note: During early stages of development, the pleural cavities containing the lung buds are located dorsally and both structures are quite small but as differentiation of the lung progresses, the pleural cavities must enlarge to accommodate the rapidly expanding lungs. Enlargement of the pleural cavities occurs by excavation and extension into the body wall and in the process, the innerface of the somatopleura is split away to produce the membranes (mediastinal pleura and pericardium) separating the heart and lungs of the adult. It is this lateral and ventral extension of the lungs and pleural cavities within the body wall that allows these structures to eventually become the most anterior visceral structures in the thorax.

Developmental Defects.   Abnormalities involving the upper respiratory passages are primarily those related to facial and oral cavity development, e.g., cleft palate. The most common developmental defects of the lower respiratory passages are those associated with defective formation of the tracheoesophageal septum, i.e., stenotic, atretic and/or fistulous lesions of the trachea and esophagus. The most important defect of the lung proper is congenital bronchial cyst; bronchial cysts may be solitary or multiple and are caused by dilation of the more distal airways. In some cases accumulation of fluid and cystic dilation appear to be related to canalization abnormalities comparable to those encountered in the digestive system.

Although prematurity is not a developmental defect, the high mortality rate in premature infants is frequently associated with respiratory problems. The single most crucial period occurs during terminal sac formation (Stage 3). In infants delivered before the 28th week, the vascularity and surface area available for gaseous exchange are usually inadequate for survival. The chances for survival increase after the 28th week but may be complicated by hyaline membrane disease or respiratory distress syndrome of the newborn. An important contributing factor in development of hyaline membrane disease is a deficiency or absence of **pulmonary surfactant**. In pregnancies with complications, lung maturation can be monitored by surfactant levels in the amniotic fluid.

QUESTIONS: Chapter 17 - Respiratory System

1. The lower portion of the respiratory system (larynx, trachea, bronchi, lungs) develops from:
   A. bilateral evaginations from the lateral wall of the foregut
   B. the caudalmost pair of pharyngeal pouches
   C. elongation and bifurcation of the thyroglossal duct
   D. a single dorsal evagination from the wall of the foregut
   E. a single ventral evagination from the wall of the foregut

2. The connective tissue, cartilage and smooth muscle of the trachea are derived from the:
   A. endoderm of the laryngotracheal groove
   B. splanchnic mesoderm of the laryngotracheal tube
   C. dermatomes of cervical somites
   D. branchiomeric mesoderm of the first branchial arch
   E. none of the above

3. Pulmonary surfactant is derived from:
   A. alveolar macrophages
   B. an ultrafiltrate of the fetal blood
   C. type I alveolar epithelial cells
   D. type II alveolar epithelial cells
   E. amniotic fluid

4. Premature infants have little chance of survival unless lung development has progressed at least as far as the stage of development referred to as the:
   A. pseudoglandular period
   B. glandular period
   C. canalicular period
   D. terminal sac period
   E. alveolar period

5. The terminal sac or 'primitive alveoli' of the developing lung are thought to be comparable to the adult:
   A. terminal bronchioles
   B. respiratory bronchioles
   C. alveolar ducts
   D. alveolar sacs
   E. none of the above

6. Defective development of the tracheoesophageal septum may lead to all of the following malformations EXCEPT:
   A. cleft palate
   B. tracheal stenosis
   C. tracheoesophageal fistula
   D. tracheal atresia
   E. esophageal atresia

Answers: 1=E; 2=B; 3=D; 4=D; 5=C; 6=A

CHAPTER 18: UROGENITAL SYSTEM

The urinary system develops from the **intermediate mesoderm** (nephrotome) connecting the segmented and nonsegmented (lateral plate) mesoderm. The genital system (gonads and genital ducts) also develop from intermediate mesoderm but the primordial germ cells originate in the yolk sac and subsequently migrate to populate the developing gonads.

Originally, both urinary and genital ducts open into the cloaca with the terminal part of the digestive system. However, after formation of the urorectal septum or fold and division of the cloaca, the urinary and genital ducts terminate in the dorsal wall of the urogenital sinus.

URINARY SYSTEM

In all mammals, three different urinary structures (pronephros, mesonephros, metanephros) are formed during the course of early development; each urinary structure is comprised of a series of **urinary tubules** joined to excretory **urinary ducts** terminating in the cloacal portion of the hindgut.

PRONEPHRIC KIDNEY

The pronephros develops at cervical levels and is the first to appear; it is very rudimentary in placental mammals.

Pronephric tubules degenerate without a trace and are so transitory in humans that they do not appear to develop in all human embryos.

Pronephric ducts degenerate cranially but persist at lower levels to serve as excretory ducts for the more caudally located mesonephric tubules, i.e., they become the mesonephric ducts.

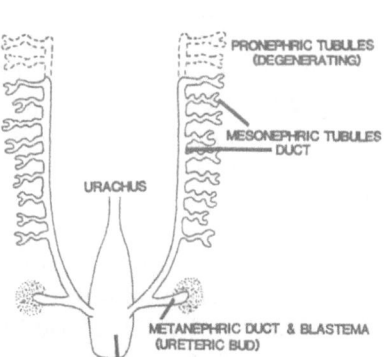

PRO, MESO, & METANEPHROS

PRONEPHRIC TUBULES (DEGENERATING)

MESONEPHRIC TUBULES — DUCT

URACHUS

METANEPHRIC DUCT & BLASTEMA (URETERIC BUD)

CLOACA

MESONEPHRIC KIDNEY

The mesonephros is very well developed but regresses without making direct contributions to the definitive urinary system. The mesonephros does, however, make direct (males) and indirect (females) contributions to the genital duct portions of the reproductive system.

Note: It is important to remember that in **all** embryos, the **mesonephric ducts** induce the formation of **paramesonephric** or **Müllerian ducts** from the adjacent coelomic epithelium. The fate of the mesonephric and paramesonephric ducts depends on the presence or absence of a hormone and a growth factor produced by the testes. Males utilize the mesonephric and females the paramesonephric ducts.

Females.   The mesonephric tubules and ducts regress without making direct contributions to either the urinary or genital systems.

Males.   Most of the mesonephric tubules regress but a few persist to form the **efferent ductules** (vasa efferentia) of the male genital system; the mesonephric duct persists to form the **ductus epididymis, ductus deferens, seminal vesicle** and **ejaculatory duct** of the genital system.

METANEPHRIC KIDNEY

The metanephros or definitive kidney has the same developmental history in both males and females. Developmentally, the **metanephric duct** (ureteric bud) appears long before the **metanephric tubules** (nephrons) begin their differentiation.

Metanephric ducts or **ureteric buds** develop as tubular outgrowths from the terminal part of the mesonephric ducts. As the ureteric buds grow dorsally and cranially, condensations of mesenchymal cells, referred to as the **metanephrogenic blastema**, collect around their distal ends. The blastemal cells will eventually differentiate to form the **metanephric tubules** or definitive **nephrons**. During subsequent development, the distal end of each ureteric bud will expand and undergo repeated divisions to form the **pelvis, major calyces, minor calyces** and **collecting ducts**, up to and including the **arched collecting tubules**, for each nephron.

DEFINITIVE KIDNEY

MINOR CALYX
MAJOR CALYX
PELVIS

URETER

Metanephric tubules or **nephrons** develop from the metanephrogenic blastemal cells associated with each terminal division of the ureteric bud. The upper end of each differentiating tubule becomes invaginated by a vascular tuft (**glomerulus**) to form the visceral (**podocyte**) and parietal layers of **Bowman's capsule**; the lower end of each developing nephron establishes continuity with a terminal division of the ureteric bud, i.e., arched collecting tubule. Nephron differentiation begins during early fetal life; at birth, the most superficial nephrons of the renal cortex have appeared but are not fully differentiated. The **renal capsule** develops from the residual cells of the metanephrogenic blastema.

Developmental Defects. It is important to emphasize that with each division of the ureteric bud there is a corresponding division of the metanephrogenic blastema; this assures that each terminal division of the ureteric bud (arched collecting tubule) possesses blastemal cells for the formation of its associated nephron (metanephric tubule). This epithelial/mesenchymal interaction explains the histological organization of the lobes (pyramids) and lobules in the adult kidney. The relationship between blastema and ureteric bud also explains why early division of the ureteric bud (partial or complete duplication of the ureter) is commonly associated with supernumerary kidneys. Horseshoe kidneys are produced by displaced ureteric buds with fusion of their associated blastemas. Blastemal fusion prevents normal rotation of the kidney and as a consequence the ureter and pelves are directed anteriorly rather than medially; blastemal fusion may also interfere with ascent of the kidneys above the level of the inferior mesenteric artery. Inadequate growth of the ureteric bud in a cranial direction may result in an ectopic kidney. Although most ectopic kidneys function normally, serious problems may arise in pregnant women with ectopic pelvic kidneys. Renal agenesis (unilateral or complete) results when ureteric buds fail to appear. The absence of ureteric buds may originate either with the formation of the bud itself or with the absence of its source of origin, i.e., the mesonephric duct. In the latter situation (absence of a mesonephric duct), the renal agenesis is frequently associated with agenesis of the genital ducts (paramesonephric as well as the mesonephric) on the affected side. Failure of the developing nephrons to establish continuity with the arched collecting tubules is thought to contribute to some types of polycystic kidney.

FORMATION OF THE URINARY BLADDER

The urinary bladder is formed from the cephalic portion of the urogenital sinus which has retained its connection to the urachal portion of the allantois. During subsequent development, the terminal portion of the mesonephric duct with its attached ureteric bud is incorporated into the wall of the urogenital sinus (trigone area). In males, the incorporation occurs in such a way that the ureteric bud terminates in the upper or urinary portion of the sinus with the mesonephric duct (vas deferens) opening into the lower or genital (prostatic) portion of the sinus. A comparable incorporation occurs in the female, but it is the terminal portion of the fused Müllerian (paramesonephric) ducts which become associated with the genital portion of the sinus.

Developmental Defects. Most developmental defects of the urinary bladder originate with abnormal partitioning of the cloacal portion of the hindgut, i.e., formation of the urorectal septum or fold. Failure of the urorectal septum to form and fuse with the cloacal membrane results in persistent cloaca; defective formation may result in various types of fistulous connections between the rectum and urinary bladder. Displacement of the urorectal septum with disproportionate division of the cloaca may result in abnormal terminations of the ureters and/or genital ducts. The persistence of a canalized urachus may result in fistulous connections between the bladder and umbilicus. Exstrophy of the bladder is the most severe developmental defect associated with bladder formation; in this condition, the anterior body and bladder walls are missing and the mucosal surface of the posterior bladder wall is exposed externally. Exstrophy of the bladder is frequently associated with musculoskeletal defects of the pelvic girdle (symphysis area) and with epispadias. This severe defect appears to originate very early and is attributed to failure of the embryonic mesoderm to fuse caudal to the cloacal membrane.

THE REPRODUCTIVE SYSTEM

Although genetic sex (XX or XY) and gonadal type (ovary or testis) are determined at the time of fertilization, it is very difficult (even microscopically) to determine the sex of a developing embryo until the early weeks of fetal development. Prior to this time, the embryo is said to be **'sexually indifferent'** because every embryo possesses:

1. the primordia for both **male** and **female genital ducts**, i.e., mesonephric and Müllerian (paramesonephric) ducts and

2. a **pudendal primordium** (genital tubercle and labioscrotal swellings) which can form either male or female genitalia.

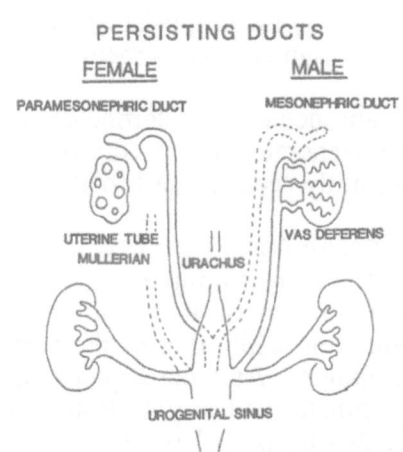

The determining factor in whether these 'indifferent primordia' differentiate as male or female genital structures **is the presence of a testis** and unless the course of differentiation is altered by testosterone stimulation, the 'indifferent primordia' of the embryo will form the accessory reproductive organs of a female; androgen production begins during the seventh week.

Differentiation of genital ducts and external genitalia in females **does not** require hormonal stimulation and will occur in the absence of ovaries.

DIFFERENTIATION OF GENITAL DUCT PRIMORDIA

The endocrine portion of the embryonic testis becomes functional during the seventh week of development and produces two substances which cause the indifferent genital duct and pudendal primordia to differentiate into those of a male.

1.   **Müllerian Inhibiting Substance** (a nonsteroidal secretion produced by the Sertoli cells of the embryonic seminiferous tubules)

2.   **Testosterone** (an androgenic steroid produced by the embryonic interstitial cells of Leydig)

The appropriate masculinizing responses in the immediately adjacent genital duct primordia (mesonephric and paramesonephric ducts) are assured by the drainage of testicular blood through the mesonephros before the testicular secretions are diluted by entering the general circulation.   Note that these are local masculinizing effects of testosterone on mesonephric derivatives only (tubules and ducts).

FATE OF THE GENITAL DUCT PRIMORDIA

Males.   The presence of testosterone stimulates the growth and development of the male primordia (mesonephric tubules and ducts) and assures development of the appropriate genital ducts for a testis (efferent ductules, ductus epididymis, ductus deferens, seminal vesicles, ejaculatory ducts).

The presence of Müllerian Inhibiting Substance causes the female primordia (Müllerian or paramesonephric ducts) to degenerate; this is why remnants of the female genital ducts are rare in normal males.

Females.   The absence of Müllerian Inhibiting Substance allows the female primordia (paramesonephric ducts) to persist and differentiate as the definitive genital ducts.   The upper ends of the ducts persist as the **uterine tubes**; the lower ends fuse to form the **uterus** and to induce vaginal development.

The absence of testosterone causes growth and development of the male primordia to cease but not degenerate; this is why remnants of the male genital ducts (Gartner's cysts and ducts) are commonly seen in the broad ligament and vaginal wall of normal females.

Developmental Defects.   Although developmental defects involving the genital ducts alone are relatively unimportant, they occur more frequently in males than in females because differentiation of the male reproductive system requires a functional gonad and hormonal stimulation while that of the female will differentiate normally without an ovary or hormonal stimulation.   As a consequence of the hormonal dependency in males, any defect in either the biosynthetic pathway of testosterone or in the expression of its masculinizing effects will be reflected by partial or complete feminization, i.e., incomplete virilization of the genital ducts and/or external genitalia.   It must be emphasized that masculinization of the genital duct primordia (mesonephric ducts) is produced by testosterone and that its masculinizing effect occurs locally, i.e., before dilution.   This localized action explains why unilateral absence of the testis during early development commonly results in an individual with rudimentary female genital ducts on the affected side and normal male ducts on the side with the testis. Developmental anomalies of this type suggest that after the testicular secretions are diluted by entering the general circulation, the levels are too low to stimulate or suppress genital duct differentiation on the opposite side.   These individuals may also exhibit feminization (ambiguous external genitalia) because the amount of testosterone produced by a single embryonic testis may be inadequate for complete masculinization of the pudendal primordium. Abnormalities in the external genitalia are more easily detected and important (medically and psychologically) than those affecting the genital ducts alone.

FORMATION OF THE VAGINA AND PROSTATIC UTRICLE

Vagina. After the caudal ends of the Müllerian ducts fuse to form the **uterus,** caudal growth brings the lower portion of the fused genital ducts into contact with the dorsal aspect of the urogenital sinus. Contact between the fused portions of the genital ducts and the urogenital sinus induces the formation of the **sinovaginal plate** or bulb which represents the primordium of the **vagina.** The vagina appears to develop as a solid epithelial proliferation from the sinovaginal plate; subsequent canalization of the epithelial outgrowth produces the **vaginal lumen.** Extension of the vaginal lumen proximally and distally establishes continuity between the cavities of the uterus and the urogenital sinus. The **hymen** is thought to mark the junctional area between the sinovaginal plate and the urogenital sinus proper, i.e., vestibule. If this interpretation is correct, the mucosal epithelium of the vagina is derived from the endoderm of the urogenital sinus and the junction between Müllerian mesoderm and vaginal endoderm would occur somewhere in the region of the **cervix.**

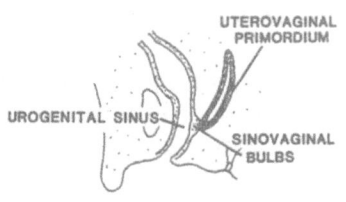

DEVELOPMENT OF THE VAGINA

UTEROVAGINAL PRIMORDIUM

UROGENITAL SINUS

SINOVAGINAL BULBS

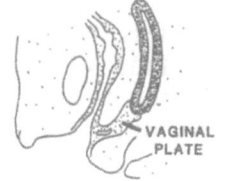

VAGINAL PLATE

Prostatic Utricle. At the present time, the **prostatic utricle** is considered to be the homologue of the female vagina. If the current interpretation of vaginal induction in the female is correct, it can be assumed that in males, the lower ends of the Müllerian ducts persist long enough to induce the formation of a sinovaginal plate for formation of the prostatic utricle.

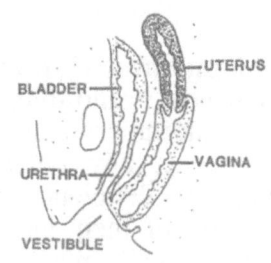

UTERUS

BLADDER

URETHRA

VAGINA

VESTIBULE

As with the genital ducts proper (mesonephric and paramesonephric), any defect in testicular function (hormone synthesis or expression) will be reflected by better development of the sinovaginal plate with a more prominent prostatic utricle (rudimentary vagina).

DIFFERENTIATION OF THE PUDENDAL PRIMORDIUM

In distal body areas, e.g., pudendal primordium, the appropriate masculinizing response in androgen sensitive cells is assured by the appearance of an enzyme (5-alpha reductase) which converts testosterone to **dihydrotestosterone;** the latter androgenic steroid is approximately fifty times more potent than testosterone. Increased potency of dihydrotestosterone compensates for the dilutional effects resulting from a small embryonic testis and a relatively large circulating blood volume (embryonic plus placental). Despite its increased potency, dihydrotestosterone cannot replace the local effects of testosterone because the mesonephric primordia (mesonephric tubules and ducts) lack the appropriate cytoplasmic receptors for dihydrotestosterone.

Note: The basic or working principles applied to differentiation of the male reproductive system are:

testosterone mediates masculinization of mesonephric derivatives (tubules and ducts) of the male genital ducts (efferent ductules, epididymal and ejaculatory ducts, seminal vesicles).

dihydrotestosterone mediates masculization of urogenital sinus derivatives (prostate, prostatic utricle and bulbourethral glands) and external genitalia (penis and scrotum).

FATE OF THE PUDENDAL PRIMORDIUM

Males. Androgenic stimulation of the indifferent pudendal primordium produces masculinization by causing greater development of the genital tubercle and by promoting fusion of the labioscrotal swellings and urethral folds, i.e., **penis, scrotum** and **penile** urethra formation.

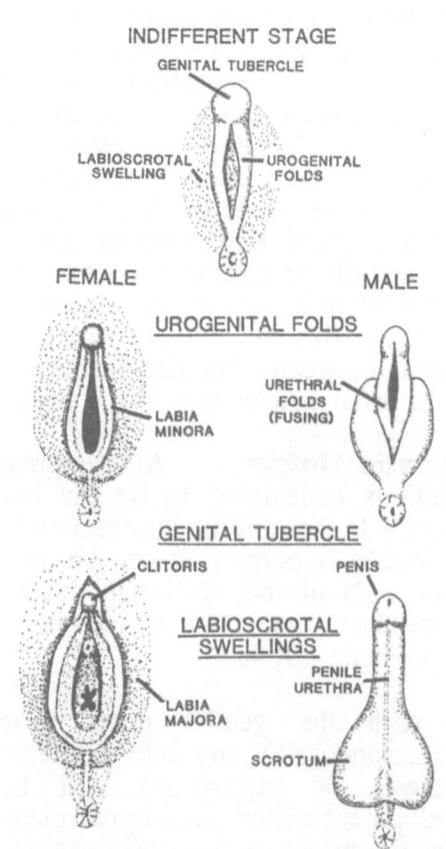

Females. The absence of androgenic stimulation results in less development of the genital tubercle and in failure of the labioscrotal swellings and urethral folds to fuse, i.e., **clitoris, labia majora** and **labia minor** formation.

Note: It must be emphasized that females also possess the enzyme 5-alpha reductase but that normally, masculinization does not occur because there is no testosterone to potentiate.

Developmental Defects. Masculinization of the pudendal primordium requires both testosterone (as a prohormone) and dihydrotestosterone. As a consequence, any defect in the biosynthesis of either, e.g., deficiency of the reductase, or in the expression of their masculinizing effects (lack of receptors) will result in partial or complete feminization of the pudendal primordium, i.e., ambiguous genitalia.

Male pseudohermaphrodites are classic examples of individuals with ambiguous genitalia due to incomplete masculinization (partial feminization). The range of ambiguity varies from forms resembling perineal hypospadias to those requiring cytogenetic analysis to determine genetic sex.

An interesting example of complete feminization is provided by individuals with **testicular feminization syndrome**. These individuals are genetic males, with normal or above normal androgen levels; masculinization fails to occur because the peripheral tissues lack androgen receptors, i.e., the defect occurs at the expression level.

Female pseudohermaphrodites are relatively rare but may be produced when female embryos are exposed to androgenic or potentially androgenic substances. The source of the androgens may be endogenous or exogenous. The best example of female pseudohermaphrodites originating from endogenous androgens is seen in individuals with **adrenogenital syndrome** (congenital virilizing adrenal hyperplasia). In this syndrome, the endogenous androgenic substances originate from the adrenal cortex and their production in excessive amounts is attributed to the high levels of ACTH resulting from a defect in cortisol biosynthesis. The virilizing effects are caused by the accumulation of cortisol precursors which are potential androgens, e.g., progesterone, and by the overproduction of weak androgens (dehydroepiandrosterone). Female pseudohermaphrodites may also occur when exogenous androgenic substances, e.g., progesterone, are administered to the mother during pregnancy; the masculinizing effects of progestins are similar to those produced by the adrenogenital syndrome.

Questions: Chapter 18 - Urogenital System

1. Bilateral renal agenesis results in:
    A. polyhydramnios
    B. premature birth
    C. increased levels of α-fetoprotein in the amniotic fluid
    D. oligohydramnios
    E. maldevelopment of the mesonephric duct

2. Which of the following urinary structures does not develop from the metanephrogenic blastema?
    A. Bowman's capsule
    B. podocytes
    C. convoluted tubules
    D. collecting tubules
    E. loop of Henle

3. Urinary function is usually absent or seriously impaired in:
    A. horseshoe kidneys
    B. ectopic kidneys
    C. pelvic kidneys
    D. supernumerary kidneys
    E. none of the above

4. Choose the **INCORRECT** statement concerning development of the genital ducts.
    A. The vagina and prostatic utricle are usually considered to be homologous structures.
    B. The pronephric ducts persist at caudal levels as the mesonephric ducts.
    C. Mesonephric ducts induce the formation of paramesonephric ducts in all embryos.
    D. Differentiation of the female genital ducts is estrogen dependent.
    E. Differentiation of the male genital ducts is testosterone dependent.

5. Accessory reproductive structures originating from the mesonephric duct include the:
    A. prostate
    B. greater vestibular glands
    C. bulbourethral glands
    D. seminal vesicles
    E. all of the above

6. Exstrophy of the bladder (ectopia vesicae) is often associated with:
    A. adrenal hyperplasia
    B. hypospadias
    C. epispadias
    D. chromosome abnormalities
    E. all of the above

Answers: 1=D; 2=D; 3=E; 4=D; 5=D; 6=C

CHAPTER 19: CARDIOVASCULAR SYSTEM

The cardiovascular system (heart, vessels, blood cells) begins to form during the third week of development. At the beginning of the fourth week (22 days), a primitive 'ebb and flow' circulation has been established; by the end of the fourth week (28 days), the blood has begun to circulate, regularly and unidirectionally, through the embryonic and extraembryonic (placental) vessels.

The initial stages in the development of the cardiovascular system, i.e., blood vessel formation (angiogenesis), are first seen in extraembryonic structures and occur almost simultaneously in the extraembryonic mesoderm of the yolk sac, body stalk and chorion; angiogenesis begins in the embryonic mesoderm a day or two later. Eventually, three separate but interdependent circulatory pathways are formed and remain functional throughout intrauterine life. Although the propulsive force (heart) and the origin of their arterial vessels (dorsal aorta) are common to all three, the vessels for

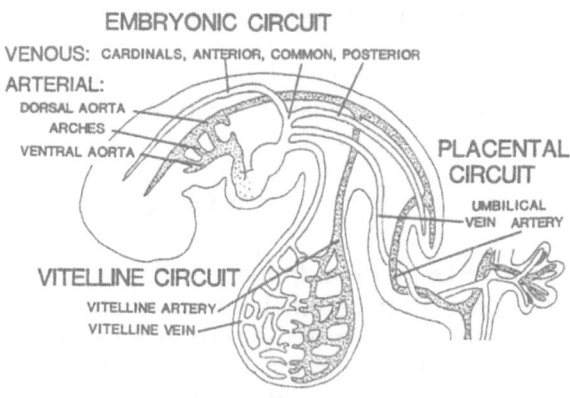

EMBRYONIC VASCULAR CIRCUITS

venous return are almost completely separated until they terminate at the venous end of the heart. The following vessels return blood from each of these circuits.

1. **cardinal veins** (anterior, posterior, common) return blood from the embryonic somatopleure or body wall area
2. **vitelline veins** return blood from both the embryonic and extraembryonic splanchnopleure, i.e., gut and yolk sac respectively
3. **umbilical (allantoic) veins** return oxygenated extraembryonic blood from the chorion

Within the embryo proper, **angiogenesis** begins in the splanchnic mesoderm forming the floor of the horseshoe shaped coelomic cavity, i.e., the cardiogenic area. The paired vessels or 'heart tubes' which develop in the cardiogenic area will subsequently fuse to form the single, midline tubular heart. Almost simultaneously a second pair of tubular vessels (primitive dorsal aortae) begins to develop on either side of the embryonic axis to establish the following arterial connections.

1. **caudally** with the extraembryonic vessels developing in the yolk sac and body stalk-chorion (placenta)
2. **cranially** with the vessels developing in the cardiogenic area ('heart tubes')

As the **paired dorsal aortae** extend cranially on either side of the oropharyngeal membrane, they anastomose with the adjacent ends of the 'heart tubes' to establish the arterial end of the heart. At the same time, the venous components of the extraembryonic vessels developing in the yolk sac (vitelline) and body stalk-chorion (umbilical or placental) establish connections with the ends of the 'heart tubes' adjacent to the septum transversum to establish the venous end of the heart.

Note: The cardinal veins which drain the body wall (somatopleure) of the embryo have not formed at this time. Their development coincides with the development of somites which are just beginning to appear. When they develop a short time later, the common cardinal veins (ducts of Cuvier) will also terminate in the septal or venous end of the heart.

During head fold formation, the arterial-venous **polarity of the heart** is reversed as the splanchnic mesoderm of the cardiogenic area and the adjacent endoderm of the yolk sac roof become incorporated into the floor of the foregut. The formation of the head fold is also responsible for the 'bend' in the primitive paired dorsal aortae which produces the first pair of **aortic arches** and the primitive paired **ventral aortae**.

The definitive positional relationships of the heart, foregut and diaphragm (septum transversum), as well as their associated coelomic derivatives, are attained when head fold formation is complete.

DEVELOPMENT OF THE HEART

The heart, like all other blood vessels, appears first as a simple **endothelial tube.** (In this case, "endo" refers to the epithelium lining all parts of the cardiovascular system **not** endoderm; all vascular elements are derived from mesoderm (endothelium, blood cells, cardiac and smooth muscle). In the definitive heart, the endothelium forming the 'heart tubes' persists as the epithelial layer of the **endocardium**; the cardiac muscle of the **myocardium** develops from splanchnic mesoderm. After the 180° rotation of the cardiogenic area which accompanies head fold formation, the heart is suspended in the pericardial cavity by a dorsal mesentery **(mesocardium).** A short time later, degeneration of the central portion of the mesocardium leaves the heart attached only at its cranial (arterial) and caudal (venous or septal) ends. The intermediate area now devoid of mesentery persists as the **transverse sinus** of the adult pericardial cavity.

DIFFERENTIATION OF THE TUBULAR HEART

The appearance of regional dilatations or expansions in the tubular heart subdivides the heart into four primitive cardiac chambers.

1. **sinus venosus** or most caudal region of the heart which receives all of the blood being returned to the heart from the three interdependent circuits
   a) common cardinal veins returning blood from the somatopleure (body wall) of the embryo
   b) vitelline or omphalomesenteric veins returning blood from the splanchnopleure (gut and yolk sac)
   c) umbilical (allantoic) veins returning blood from the placenta
2. **primitive atrium**
3. **primitive ventricle**
4. **bulbus cordis** and **truncus arteriosus** which form the most cranial portion of the heart (The truncus arteriosus represents the fused portions of the primitive ventral aortae; the unfused portions are continued cranially and dorsally as the first pair of aortic arches.)

The tubular heart, anchored at its cranial and caudal ends, elongates more rapidly than the surrounding pericardial cavity and subsequently bends ventrally and to the right side of the pericardial cavity. With increased growth, the ventricular and bulbar regions come to lie immediately adjacent to each other. As a consequence of these growth changes, the bulbar portion becomes pressed against the more dorsally situated atrial area. As the atrial region enlarges, it expands on either side of the bulbus producing the primordia of the future right and left atrial chambers. The subsequent fate for each of the four regions of the primitive heart are summarized below.

1. The **primitive atrium** becomes divided into right and left atria and the sinus venosus becomes incorporated into the definitive right atrium.

2. The **primitive ventricle** forms all of the left ventricle of the adult heart except the outflow area of the aorta.

3. The **bulbus cordis** forms all of the right ventricle including the pulmonary outflow area and the aortic outflow area of the left ventricle.

4. The **truncus arteriosus** (ventral aorta) becomes partitioned to form the origin for the aorta and for the pulmonary artery.

PRIMITIVE HEART TUBE

Fate of the Sinus Venosus. All venous blood returning to the heart flows into the sinus venosus through three pairs of veins (common cardinals, vitelline, umbilical). Very early the sinus venosus is located within the septum transversum, but as the heart enlarges the sinus venosus appears to be "pulled out" of the septum and into the pericardial cavity. It is important to remember that all of the veins listed above pass through the septum transversum to reach the heart. This is particularly important with respect to the fate of the vitelline (omphalomesenteric) and umbilical veins and their relationship to the developing liver which proliferates within the septum transversum.

Initially, the opening between the sinus venosus and the primitive atrium is located in the midline but as venous blood is shunted to the right side of the heart, the right extremity of the sinus venosus (right horn) enlarges moving the sinoatrial opening to the right. Later, the right horn of the sinus venosus becomes incorporated into the primitive atrium to form the **smooth portion** of the definitive right atrium; the right half of the primitive atrium possesses **musculi pectinati** and persists as the **right auricular appendage**. The left horn of the sinus venosus remains small because venous return is being shifted to the right side of the heart; it persists in the adult as the **coronary sinus** and receives only venous blood from the heart itself.

Fate of the Primitive Pulmonary Veins. The earliest stages in the development of the pulmonary veins is controversial but despite the uncertainty concerning their precise origin, once they are present, the terminal portion is incorporated into the left half of the primitive atrium to form the **smooth portion** of the left atrium; the left half of the primitive atrium possesses **musculi pectinati** and persists as the **left auricular appendage**. Resorption of the primitive pulmonary vessels extends distally to the appropriate bifurcation level to produce the four definitive pulmonary veins of the adult heart. The **oblique sinus** of the pericardial cavity is formed by pericardial reflections surrounding pulmonary veins and venae cavae, i.e., the pericardial reflection surrounding the venous end of the heart.

DEVELOPMENT OF THE FOUR CHAMBERED HEART

As the tubular heart changes shape and position, a series of septa develop which convert the folded tubular heart into the four chambers recognized in the adult heart. It is important to realize that all of the changes occurring in the developing cardiovascular system, heart and vessels, are taking place simultaneously and are presented separately only for simplicity. It should also be emphasized that all of these changes occur without interrupting the continuous pumping action of the heart.

DIVISION OF THE COMMON ATRIOVENTRICULAR OPENING

Localized proliferations of mesenchyme within the anterior and posterior walls of the common atrioventricular opening are responsible for the appearance of two elevations which are referred to as the **endocardial cushions**. Subsequent growth and fusion of the dorsal and ventral endocardial cushions divides the common atrioventricular opening into definitive **right** (tricuspid) and **left** (mitral) **atrioventricular canals**. A short time later, the fused endocardial cushions will also participate in effecting complete separation of the definitive atria and ventricles by contributing to the formation of the interatrial (septum primum) and interventricular (membranous portion) septa.

DIVISION OF COMMON A / V CANAL

Developmental Defects. Cardiac anomalies, which include a common atrioventricular canal, narrowing (stenosis) or widening (dilatation) of either the right (tricuspid) or left (mitral) atrioventricular canals, interatrial septal defects involving the septum primum, or high interventricular septal defects as one of their components, may have their developmental origin at this stage of cardiac development.

Persistence of the common or primitive A/V opening is caused by failure of the endocardial cushions to fuse; this is one of the common cardiac defects associated with Down's syndrome. The same fusion failure of the dorsal and ventral endocardial cushions would also disrupt their subsequent fusion with the septum primum and contribute to atrial septal defects. Displacement to the right or left would produce tricuspid or mitral stenosis with dilatation of the corresponding canal on the opposite side. Displacement to either side would also dislocate its contributions to the membranous septum and contribute to high interventricular septal defects.

DEVELOPMENT OF THE CARDIAC SKELETON AND CONDUCTING SYSTEM

The four fibrous rings (annuli fibrosi) of the cardiac skeleton which surround the atrioventricular canals and the origins of the aorta and pulmonary artery will subsequently differentiate at the level of the endocardial cashions. It should be noted that these fibrous rings serve as attachment sites for the cardiac valves and as origin and insertion points for the cardiac muscle fibers of the myocardium. Eventually, the cardiac skeleton will completely separate the atrial and ventricular myocardium; in the adult heart, the atrioventricular **bundle of His** is the only direct connection between the atrial and ventricular musculature. Developmentally, the **Purkinje tissue** of the conducting system differentiates from regular cardiac muscle but it is specialized for conduction rather than contraction. Large septal defects (atrial or ventricular) may encroach on the bundle of His to produce cardiac arrhythmias (bundle block).

FORMATION OF THE INTERATRIAL SEPTUM

The formation of two septa (primum and secundum) is required to effect complete separation of the single primitive atrium into the definitive right and left atria of the adult heart.

Septum Primum. The first septum (septum I) forms as a crescentic-shaped partition and grows inferiorly to fuse with the endocardial cushions which have just joined to produce the definitive right and left A/V canals. However, before fusion between the lower part of septum I and the endocardial cushions is complete, the upper portion of septum I degenerates to produce a new opening or foramen (ostium II). The new opening or ostium II maintains the communication between the developing atria as the original foramen (ostium I) is obliterated.

Note: Ostium I is a transitory opening formed by the sickle-shaped edge of septum I; this opening is gradually obliterated as the inferior edge fuses with the endocardial cushions. Ostium I cannot be obliterated until ostium II develops to maintain the right to left venous shunt within the heart.

Septum Secundum. The second septum (septum II) is also crescentic in shape and develops immediately to the right of septum I. Septum II grows inferiorly but does **not** fuse with the endocardial cushions. The opening left by the curved inferior edge of septum II is the **foramen ovale**. The persistent, lower portion of septum I functions as the **valve of the foramen ovale**.

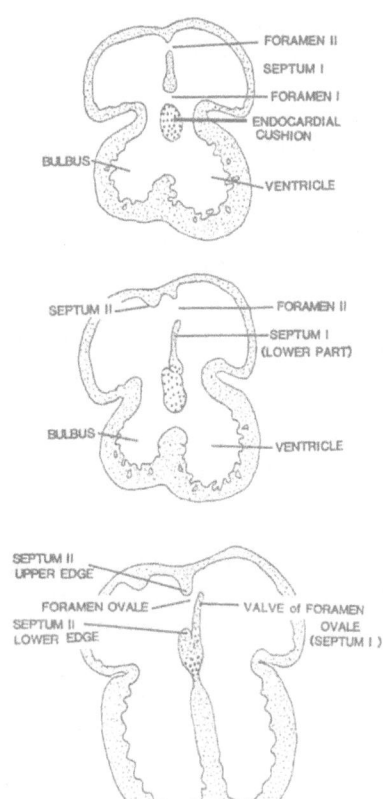

INTERATRIAL SEPTUM FORMATION

FORMATION OF THE DEFINITIVE VENTRICLES

It is important to remember that the primitive ventricle and bulbus cordis were brought into a side by side relationship by flexion of the primitive heart tube and that these two structures form the following adult structures.

1. The **primitive ventricle** forms all of the definitive left ventricle **except** the aortic outlet.
2. The **bulbus cordis** forms all of the definitive right ventricle **and** the aortic outlet of the left ventricle.

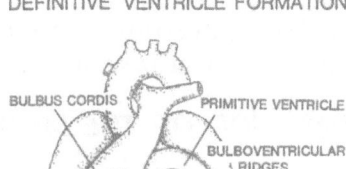

DEFINITIVE VENTRICLE FORMATION

During the final stages of flexion, the broad communication (bulboventricular canal) between the primitive ventricle and bulbus cordis is partially closed by the appearance of **superior** and **inferior bulboventricular ridges** which form the boundaries of the future interventricular foramen.

FATE OF THE BULBOVENTRICULAR RIDGES

The **superior ridge** is actually a prominent fold in the developing myocardium; it is produced during flexion when the wall of the bulbus cordis is folded against the adjacent wall of the primitive ventricle. Regression of the superior ridge brings the upper portion of the left ventricle into direct communication with arterial outflow area of the bulbus, i.e., truncus arteriosus; this is how the bulbus cordis forms the aortic outlet for the left ventricle.

The **inferior ridge** persists as the primordium for the muscular portion of the interventricular septum; its increasing prominence appears to be caused more by expansion of the adjacent ventricles than by actual growth of the septum itself.

Complete separation of the definitive right and left ventricles, i.e., closure of the interventricular foramen, is effected by the formation of the membranous part of the interventricular septum; this occurs during partitioning of the truncus arteriosus.

FORMATION OF THE AORTIC AND PULMONARY TRUNKS

FATE OF THE TRUNCUS ARTERIOSUS

DIVISION OF THE TRUNCUS

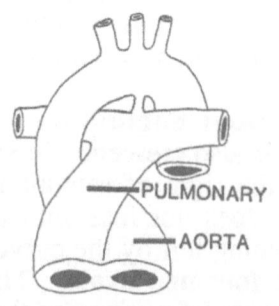

The truncus arteriosus is divided into aortic and pulmonary trunks by formation of the **aorticopulmonary** or **spiral septum**. The aorticopulmonary (spiral) septum develops from two spiraling ridges of intimal mesenchyme which project into the lumen of the truncus arteriosus; subsequent growth and fusion of the spiral ridges produce the separate lumina for the **aortic and pulmonary trunks**. Luminal division is followed by separation of the arterial walls and is responsible for the twisted configuration of the adult vessels. The distal portion of the spiral septum is strategically placed between the origins of the fourth (systemic) and sixth (pulmonary) aortic arches and assures that blood from the right ventricle is delivered to the sixth arch and that the blood from the left ventricle is delivered to the fourth arch.

Developmental Defects. Complete absence of the spiral septum results in persistent truncus; incomplete fusion of the ridges results in aorticopulmonary communications; incomplete spiraling results in transposition of the great vessels; displacement of the ridges with unequal division of the truncus results in pulmonary or aortic stenosis with dilatation of the opposite vessel. Displacement of the lower ends of the spiral ridges interferes with formation of the membranous septum and results in high interventricular septal defect, i.e., persistent interventricular foramen. The anatomical defects in the **tetralogy of Fallot** (pulmonary stenosis, septal defect, overriding aorta) are thought to arise in this way (the right ventricular hypertrophy is a physiological response to the pulmonary stenosis).

FORMATION OF THE MEMBRANOUS SEPTUM

Final closure of the interventricular foramen is accomplished by the formation of the membranous part of the interventricular septum. Its formation involves the proliferation and fusion of mesenchyme from the proximal ends of both **spiral ridges** and from the **endocardial cushions** (particularly the dorsal). Displacement of either ridge or cushion will interfere with fusion and contribute to the formation of a membranous septal defect.

MEMBRANOUS SEPTUM FORMATION

SPIRAL RIDGES

ENDOCARDIAL CUSHION

RIGHT AV CANAL

Note: Structures which develop by active growth processes and fusions are frequently attended by developmental defects when the growth process is inadequate or when fusion fails to occur. Complexity in formation provides greater chance for abnormal development. The formation of the atrial and ventricular septa is extremely complex and, consequently, both areas are frequently involved in cardiac anomalies; both are recent acquisitions from the evolutionary standpoint.

DEVELOPMENT OF THE ARTERIAL SYSTEM

AORTIC ARCHES

Each branchial arch complex contains an aortic arch which connects the dorsal and ventral (truncus arteriosus) aortae. In lower vertebrates, the aortic arches form rich vascular plexi on the surfaces of the branchial arches to produce functional gills although the respiratory function for most of the branchial arches has been lost, six aortic arches still appear during human development. Three of these persist (three, four, six) and make definitive contributions to the adult vasculature but only the sixth has retained a respiratory function. Their appearance in the human embryo is often transitory and all six are not present at the same time. The sixth or incomplete branchial arch, which is continuous with the adjacent body wall, contains a well developed aortic arch.

The contributions of aortic arches to the adult vasculature are illustrated in the accompanying diagrams.

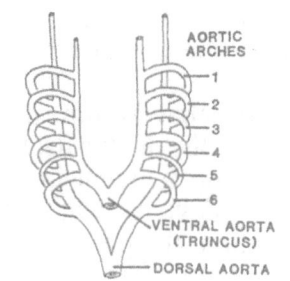

FATE OF THE AORTIC ARCHES

AORTIC ARCH 1 is the first to appear and is formed as a result of head fold formation; it disappears soon after development. The mandibular and maxillary areas of the adult are supplied by new vessels arising from the external carotid, i.e., cranial extension of the ventral aorta into the developing head region.

AORTIC ARCH 2 also persists only during the early stages of development. A small portion of this vessel, the stapedial artery, persists while the stapes is forming from Reichert's cartilage. The presence of the stapedial artery is thought to be responsible for the "y" shaped configuration of the stapes. After the artery degenerates, its original position is marked by the space between the two rami and foot plate of the stapes.

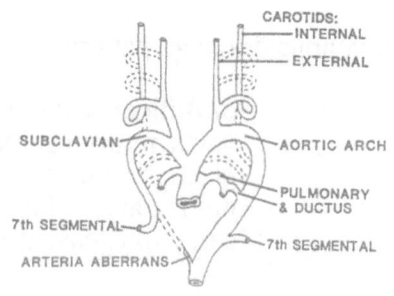

AORTIC ARCH 3 persists in the adult to form the **origin of the internal carotid artery.** **Note:** The dorsal aorta between aortic arches 3 and 4 disappears and the extension of the internal carotid into the cranial area is an active growth process of the dorsal aorta, to supply the rapidly enlarging brain.

AORTIC ARCH 4 persists on the left side as the **arch of the aorta**; on the right it contributes to the brachiocephalic artery and the proximal portion of the right subclavian artery.

AORTIC ARCH 5 is extremely transitory and does not appear to develop in all human embryos. The developmental variability appears to be related to the rudimentary condition of the fifth branchial arch.

AORTIC ARCH 6 is well developed and forms the origin or proximal portion of the pulmonary arteries; the distal portions of the pulmonary arteries arise directly from the sixth arch and accompany the developing lung buds into the pleural cavities. **Note:** On the right side the original connection of the sixth arch to the dorsal aorta is lost and the recurrent laryngeal nerve (the nerve for the branchiomeric musculature developing from the sixth arch) slips cranially to loop around the right subclavian artery (fourth arch). On the left side, the connection is retained as the **ductus arteriosus** and as a consequence the left recurrent laryngeal nerve descends into the thorax to 'recur' around the ligamentum arteriosum.

Developmental Defects.   Although the exact cause for coarctation of the aorta is not known, the narrowing usually occurs in the immediate vicinity of the ductus arteriosus. One widely held theory is that muscle tissue from vessels which normally regress (ductus arteriosus and right side of the paired dorsal aortae) is incorporated into the adjacent wall of definitive vessels and subsequent regression of the displaced muscle tissue causes narrowing of the persisting vessel.

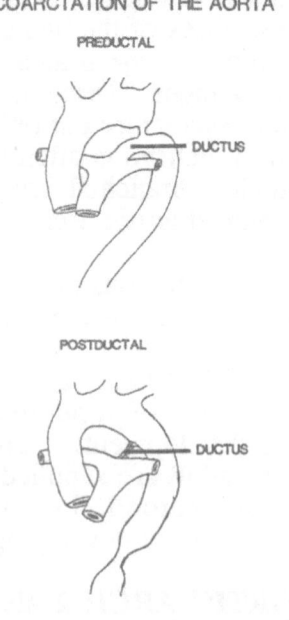

COARCTATION OF THE AORTA

PREDUCTAL

DUCTUS

POSTDUCTAL

DUCTUS

Postductal coarctation is the most common form and is usually located immediately below the origin of the left subclavian, i.e., in the area of the regressing right dorsal aorta.   Postductal coarctation probably has its origin during fetal life but, because of better collateral circulation, this form of coarctation may go undetected for years.   It is for this reason that it is sometimes referred to as the **adult form** of coarctation.

Preductal coarctations are located immediately above the ductus arteriosus; the ductus itself is almost invariable patent. The length of the aortic segment involved may be extensive and its location precludes development of collateral circulation. Without surgical intervention, the prognosis is poor. Since the condition is detected at or shortly after birth, the preductal narrowing is frequently referred to as the **infantile form** of coarctation.

DEVELOPMENT OF THE VENOUS SYSTEM

The venous drainage pattern of the early human embryo consists of the following paired veins:

1.   **umbilical** or **allantoic** (placental) veins returning blood from the placenta (these veins like the pulmonary veins of the adult, carry oxygenated blood).

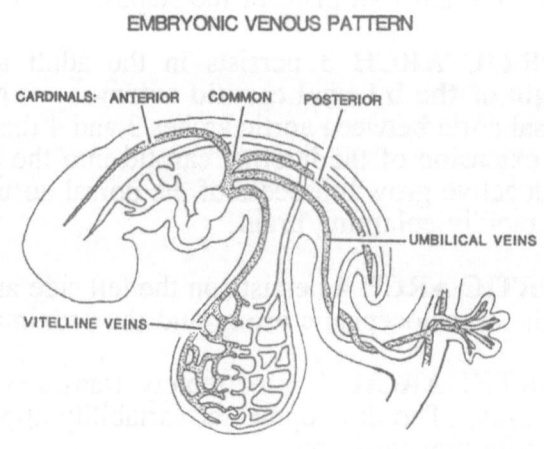

EMBRYONIC VENOUS PATTERN

CARDINALS: ANTERIOR COMMON POSTERIOR

UMBILICAL VEINS

VITELLINE VEINS

2.   **vitelline** or **omphalomesenteric** veins returning blood from the splanchnopleure, i.e., yolk sac and gut derivatives. **Note:** The definitive   pulmonary   veins appear rather late in embryonic life and are said to originate from the dorsal part of the left atrium and grow into the lung.

3.   **cardinal** (anterior, posterior, common) veins returning blood from the somatopleure of the embryo. **Note:** The anterior cardinals drain the cranial levels of the embryo (head, upper extremities), i.e., levels above the septum transversum; posterior cardinals drain levels of the embryo below the septum transversum. The terminal portions of both unite to form the common cardinals (ducts of Cuvier).

All of these vessels return blood to the fetal heart by passing through the septum transversum before terminating in the sinus venosus.

FATE OF THE UMBILICAL (ALLANTOIC) VEINS

The right umbilical vein disappears during early development leaving the left as a functional vessel until the cord is severed at parturition. In the region of the septum transversum, the developing liver surrounds the terminal part of the umbilical vein; this intrahepatic portion of the umbilical vein is the **ductus venosus**.

After birth, the extrahepatic portion becomes fibrous and persists in the adult as the **ligamentum teres hepatis**; the intrahepatic portion persists as the **ligamentum venosum**.

FATE OF THE VITELLINE VEINS

The vitelline vessels draining the splanchnopleuric (gut and yolk sac) areas of the fetus are relatively unimportant during intrauterine life because the gut is essentially nonfunctional; they are important postnatally because of their contributions to the hepatic portal system. The **hepatic portal vein** is derived in part from the extrahepatic portions of both vitelline veins and from intervenous anastomoses. The intrahepatic portions of the vitelline are invaded by hepatic cords but persist as the **hepatic sinusoids, central, sublobular** and **hepatic veins** of the adult liver.

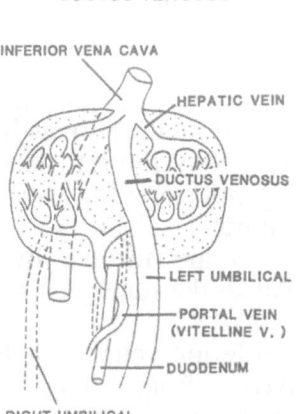

DUCTUS VENOSUS

INFERIOR VENA CAVA

HEPATIC VEIN

DUCTUS VENOSUS

LEFT UMBILICAL

PORTAL VEIN (VITELLINE V.)

DUODENUM

RIGHT UMBILICAL

Note: The cephalic portion of the vitelline system is extremely rudimentary in placental mammals, but its existence explains the unusual termination of the pulmonary veins in anomalous pulmonary venous return. In this condition, the pulmonary veins almost invariably terminate either:

1. **below the diaphragm** in hepatic or portal veins (both are derived from the vitelline system below the diaphragm, i.e., 'posterior' vitelline veins) or

2. **above the diaphragm** into veins derived from the cephalic portion of the supracardinal capillary plexus (azygos, hemiazygos, accessory hemiazygos).

The termination of pulmonary veins in azygos vessels is explained by the persistence (and enlargement) of anastomotic connections between the vitelline and supracardinal capillary networks within the short, broad, dorsal mesentery of the esophagus above the diaphragm, i.e, primitive mediastinum, anastomotic connections between the vitelline and supracardinal capillary networks are essentially nonexistent in the long, narrow, dorsal mesentery of the gut below the diaphragm.

FATE OF THE ANTERIOR, POSTERIOR AND COMMON CARDINAL VEINS

The **anterior cardinal veins** persist as the **internal jugular veins** in the adult but only the right contributes to the formation of the superior vena cava. A new vessel (left brachiocephalic) forms across the midline to shunt blood from the left anterior cardinal to the right. The terminal portion of the right anterior cardinal forms the **superior vena cava**; fibrous remnants of the left anterior cardinal persist in the adult as the **ligament of the left superior vena cava**. This ligamentous structure connects the left superior intercostal vein to the coronary sinus of the heart via the **oblique vein of the left atrium**. It should be remembered that the coronary sinus is formed from the left horn of the sinus venosus. **Note:** When the left brachiocephalic vein fails to form, the terminal portion of the left anterior cardinal remains functional and forms a left superior vena cava terminating (via the oblique veins) in the coronary sinus.

The **posterior cardinal veins** regress and are replaced by a new somatopleuric vessel, the **inferior vena cava**, which originates from capillary plexi located above and below the posterior cardinals, i.e., supracardinal and subcardinal plexi.

Note: The **supracardinals** and **subcardinals** are capillary plexi associated with the cardinal system. Although these plexi are paired, they are characterized by the richness of their anastomotic connections and especially those crossing the midline **anterior** and **posterior** to the dorsal aorta. During regression of the mesonephric kidney and posterior cardinal veins, these capillary plexi increase in prominence and begin to produce discrete venous channels which contribute to the adult vasculature, e.g., the inferior vena cava.

FORMATION OF THE INFERIOR VENA CAVA

The upper portion of the inferior vena cava, from the diaphragm to and including the renal veins, is derived from the **subcardinal** midline anastomoses. (This is why the left renal vein and upper portion of the inferior vena cava are anterior or 'sub' to the aorta.) The gonadal veins (testicular or ovarian) are formed by the subcardinal vessels caudal to the renal veins.

The inferior vena cava below the renal veins is derived from the **supracardinal** midline anastomoses. (This is why the lower part of the inferior vena cava and common iliac veins are located posterior or 'supra') to the aorta; above this level, the supracardinals form the **azygos** and **hemiazygos veins**. (This is also why the azygos vessels retain a caudal connection to the inferior vena cava.)

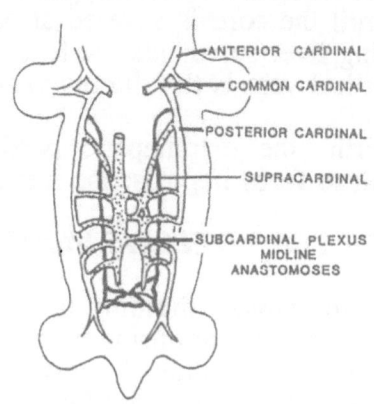

INFERIOR VENA CAVA FORMATION

- ANTERIOR CARDINAL
- COMMON CARDINAL
- POSTERIOR CARDINAL
- SUPRACARDINAL
- SUBCARDINAL PLEXUS MIDLINE ANASTOMOSES

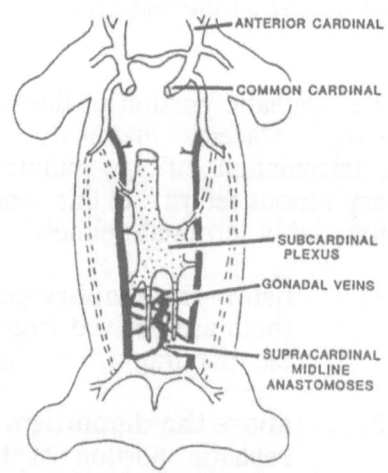

- ANTERIOR CARDINAL
- COMMON CARDINAL
- SUBCARDINAL PLEXUS
- GONADAL VEINS
- SUPRACARDINAL MIDLINE ANASTOMOSES

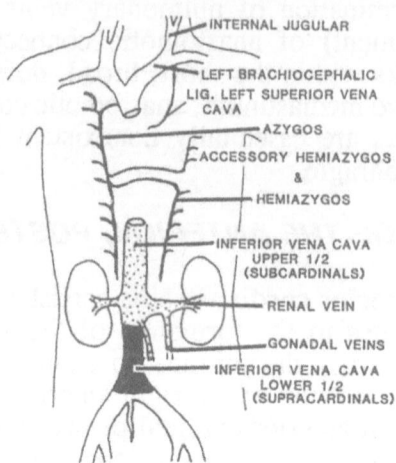

DEFINITIVE VENOUS SYSTEM

- INTERNAL JUGULAR
- LEFT BRACHIOCEPHALIC
- LIG. LEFT SUPERIOR VENA CAVA
- AZYGOS
- ACCESSORY HEMIAZYGOS & HEMIAZYGOS
- INFERIOR VENA CAVA UPPER 1/2 (SUBCARDINALS)
- RENAL VEIN
- GONADAL VEINS
- INFERIOR VENA CAVA LOWER 1/2 (SUPRACARDINALS)

QUESTIONS: Chapter 19 - Cardiovascular System

1.   The heart musculature or myocardium develops from:
      A.   splanchnic mesoderm
      B.   somatic mesoderm
      C.   branchiomeric mesenchyme
      D.   segmented mesoderm
      E.   ectomesenchyme (neural crest)

2.   The right ventricle of the definitive heart appears to be derived almost entirely from the primitive:
      A.   sinus venosus
      B.   atrium
      C.   ventricle
      D.   bulbus cordis
      E.   truncus arteriosus

3.   The coronary sinus is generally considered to be derived from the:
      A.   right horn of the sinus venosus
      B.   left horn of the sinus venosus
      C.   right common cardinal (duct of Cuvier)
      D.   terminal portion of the primitive pulmonary vein
      E.   terminal portions of the vitelline (omphalomesenteric) veins

4.   Which of the following conditions does **NOT** occur in the malformation tetralogy of Fallot?
      A.   pulmonary stenosis
      B.   large foramen ovale
      C.   right ventricular hypertrophy
      D.   dextropositional (overriding) aorta
      E.   large ventricular septal defect

5.   The aortic arches which disappear without making significant contributions to the adult vasculature are:
      A.   one, two and three
      B.   one, two and four
      C.   one, two and five
      D.   one, two and six
      E.   none of the above combinations is correct

6.   Maldevelopment of the endocardial cushions may result in:
      A.   common atrioventricular canal
      B.   interatrial septal defect involving the septum primum
      C.   stenosis of the right atrioventricular canal
      D.   high interventricular septal defect
      E.   all of the above

Answers: 1=A; 2=D; 3=B; 4=B; 5=C; 6=E

CHAPTER 20: FETAL CIRCULATION AND CHANGES AT BIRTH

FETAL CIRCULATION

Before birth, the respiratory functions of the lungs are performed by the placenta and, as a consequence, the umbilical (allantoic) or placental veins carry oxygenated blood back to the heart. Functionally, the umbilical veins of the embryo and fetus are comparable to the postnatal pulmonary veins.

During early development, the umbilical veins are paired vessels which terminate directly in the primitive tubular heart, i.e., sinus venosus. However, after subsequent developmental changes which include:

1.   development of the liver and regression of the right umbilical vein,
2.   development of the hepatic portal circulation from the vitelline veins,
3.   formation of the inferior vena cava which accompanied regression of the posterior cardinal veins, and
4.   incorporation of the sinus venosus into the definitive four chambered heart,

the oxygenated blood carried by the persisting left umbilical vein is shunted into the inferior vena cava by the ductus venosus.

Note: Within the inferior vena cava, the umbilical blood is mixed with smaller amounts of venous blood from the caudal levels of the body. Despite this mixture of oxygenated (umbilical) and unoxygenated (caval) blood, the inferior vena cava carries the most highly oxygenated blood available during development; the superior vena cava carries only deoxygenated blood.

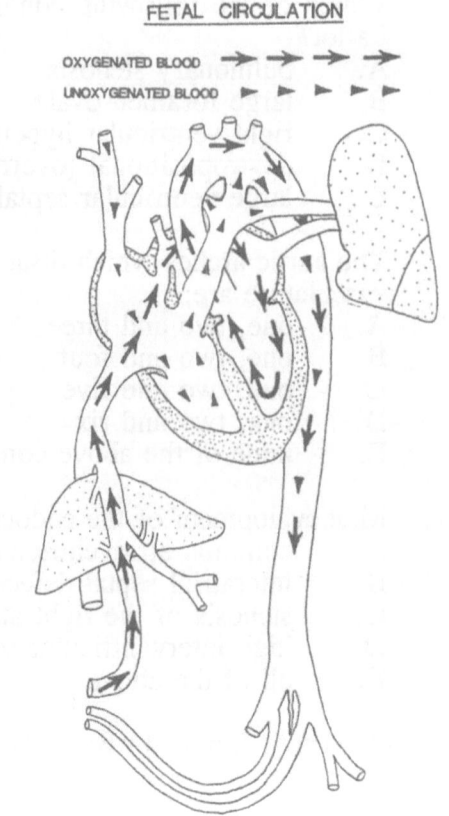

FETAL CIRCULATION

OXYGENATED BLOOD

UNOXYGENATED BLOOD

PATHWAY OF OXYGENATED BLOOD

Oxygenated blood in the inferior vena cava enters the right atrium and is diverted through the **foramen ovale** into the left atrium. The oxygenated blood then passes through the left **atrioventricular (mitral) opening** and leaves the **left ventricle** via the **ascending aorta**. From the arch of the aorta, the oxygenated blood is distributed via the brachiocephalic trunk and the left common carotid and subclavian arteries to the upper portion of the body. The intracardiac shunt via the foramen ovale assures that the head and especially the developing brain receives the most highly oxygenated blood available.

PATHWAY OF DEOXYGENATED BLOOD

Deoxygenated blood from the upper half of the body enters the right atrium from the superior vena cava and passes directly through the **right atrioventricular (tricuspid) opening** to enter the **right ventricle** and **pulmonary trunk**. A small portion of the deoxygenated blood enters the pulmonary arteries to perfuse the developing lungs but the major portion is shunted **via the ductus arteriosus** into the thoracic aorta below the origin of the left subclavian artery. All structures receiving their blood supply from arteries arising from the aorta below the origin of the left subclavian artery are perfused by a mixture of oxygenated and deoxygenated blood.

CHANGES IN THE CIRCULATION AT BIRTH

FATE OF THE FORAMEN OVALE

At birth, the right to left shunt provided by the foramen ovale ceases to function when changes in atrial pressure bring the overlapping portions of the septum primum (valve of the foramen ovale) and the septum secundum into apposition. The primary cause of septal apposition (closure of the foramen ovale) appears to be the result of an abrupt decrease in right atrial pressure which is associated with the sudden termination of placental circulation at birth, i.e., clamping or tying the umbilical cord. Apposition may also be enhanced by the increase in left atrial pressure which is associated with the onset of pulmonary function, i.e., increased perfusion and venous return.

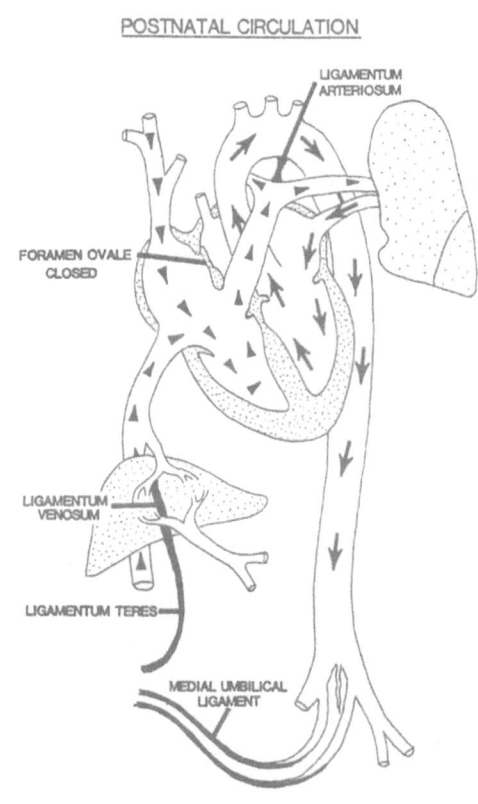

Failure of the foramen ovale to close anatomically (fusion of the septum primum and secundum) is relatively common, i.e., probe patent foramen ovale, but is insignificant physiologically. A large patent or open foramen ovale usually has its origin during embryonic life and is attributable to faulty development of the septum primum and/or the septum secundum.

In the adult heart, the location and boundaries of the foramen ovale are indicated by the **limbus fossae ovalis**; the **floor of the fossa ovalis** is formed by the septum primum.

FATE OF THE DUCTUS ARTERIOSUS

The ductus arteriosus begins to close almost immediately after birth and may be closed functionally within a few hours; complete obliteration of the lumen and fibrosis may require three or four weeks. It persists throughout life as the **ligamentum arteriosum.**

Note: In some heart anomalies, survival may depend on a patent ductus arteriosus. Closure can sometimes be prevented or delayed by prostaglandin infusions until surgery can be performed. Conversely, when patency is undesirable, inhibition of prostaglandin synthesis, e.g., indomethacin, can sometimes be used to induce closure without surgery.

FATE OF THE UMBILICAL VEIN AND DUCTUS VENOSUS

After interruption of the placental circulation, the extra- and intrahepatic portions of the umbilical vein become reduced to fibrotic cords which persist in the adult as the **ligamentum** teres hepatis and ligamentum venosum respectively.

FATE OF THE UMBILICAL ARTERIES

In the adult, the proximal portions of the umbilical arteries persist as the umbilical branches of the internal iliacs; the distal portions which accompany the intraembryonic portion of the allantois (urachus) are obliterated but persist as the **medial umbilical ligaments**; the urachus itself persists as the **median umbilical ligament**.

QUESTIONS: Chapter 20 - Fetal Circulation

1. The ductus arteriosus is formed by a portion of aortic arch:
   A. four on the left side
   B. four on the right side
   C. six on the left side
   D. six on the right side
   E. six from both sides

2. Oxygenated blood mixes with deoxygenated blood in the developing fetus in the:
   A. descending aorta
   B. right atrium
   C. liver
   D. inferior vena cava
   E. all of the above

3. Adult structures derived from fetal blood vessels include all of the following **EXCEPT** the:
   A. median umbilical ligament
   B. medial umbilical ligaments
   C. ligamentum teres hepatis
   D. ligamentum venosum
   E. ligamentum arteriosum

4. Choose the **CORRECT** statement concerning coarctation of the aorta.
   A. Preductal coarctation is usually associated with a patent ductus arteriosus.
   B. Preductal coarctation is usually detected at or shortly after birth.
   C. Preductal coarctation usually has a poor prognosis without surgical intervention.
   D. Collateral circulation may allow postductal coarctation to go undetected for years.
   E. All of the above statements are true.

5. Umbilical arteries carry:
   A. deoxygenated blood to the placenta
   B. oxygenated blood to the placenta
   C. oxygenated blood to the embryo
   D. deoxygenated blood to the embryo
   E. deoxygenated blood through the liver

6. The oblique vein of the left atrium represents part of the:
   A. anterior cardinal system
   B. supracardinal system
   C. subcardical system
   D. vitelline system
   E. none of the above

Answers: 1=C; 2=E; 3=A; 4=E; 5=A; 6=A